Acupressure
for
Emotional Healing

Other Self-Care Resources*
by Michael Reed Gach, PhD

BOOKS
- Acu-Yoga
- Acupressure's Potent Points
- Acupressure for Lovers
- Arthritis Relief at Your Fingertips

BOOKLETS
- Acu–Face Lift
- Acupressure Weight Loss
- Acupressure for Health Professionals
- Hand & Foot Reflexology
- Introduction to Acupressure
- Meridians, Five Elements & Assessment Forms
- Shiatsu Course Workbook
- Traditional Thai Massage

GUIDED SELF-HEALING CDs
- Sleep Better
- Stress Relief
- Increase Vitality
- Release Back Pain

INSTRUCTIONAL VIDEOS
- Acupressure Stress Relief
- Bum Back Video
- Emotional Healing Video
- Fundamentals of Acupressure
- Releasing Shoulder & Neck Tension
- Stress-Less Breathing Exercises
- Zen Shiatsu Instruction

ACUPRESSURE POINT CHART
Includes a Self-Care Point Recipe Booklet

*See Appendix D at the back of the book for more information to obtain these self-care resources.

Acupressure for Emotional Healing

A Self-Care Guide for Trauma,
Stress & Common Emotional Imbalances

Michael Reed Gach, PhD
Author of Acupressure's Potent Points

Beth Ann Henning, Dipl ABT

BANTAM BOOKS
NEW YORK • TORONTO • LONDON • SYDNEY • AUCKLAND

ACUPRESSURE FOR EMOTIONAL HEALING
A Bantam Book / November 2004

Published by
Bantam Dell
A Division of Random House, Inc.
New York, New York

Library of Congress Cataloging-in-Publication Data

Gach, Michael Reed.
    Acupressure for emotional healing : a self-care guide for trauma, stress and common emotional
imbalances / Michael Reed Gach, Beth Ann Henning.
        p. cm.
    Includes bibliographical references and index.
    ISBN 0-553-38243-8
    1. Acupressure—Popular works. 2. Emotions—Popular works. 3. Healing—Popular works.
4. Mind and body—Popular works. I. Henning, Beth Ann. II. Title.

    RM723.A27G328 2004
    615.8'222—dc22

                                                                2004056052

Manufactured in the United States of America
Published simultaneously in Canada

RRH 10 9 8 7 6 5 4 3 2 1

DEDICATION

*We dedicate this book to those who need
        emotional healing.
We've seen how trauma and emotional pain
        stifle the quality of life,
And how acupressure has transformed and
        healed people.*

*May this book enable you to
        heal the depths of your heart,
And provide new ways to open
        and renew your spirit.*

*May this book make emotional healing accessible,
Given the immense stress in the world.*

*Through the ancient art of acupressure,
Along with slow, deep breathing,
Emotional healing is within your reach,
Governed by the life force that flows
        through the points.*

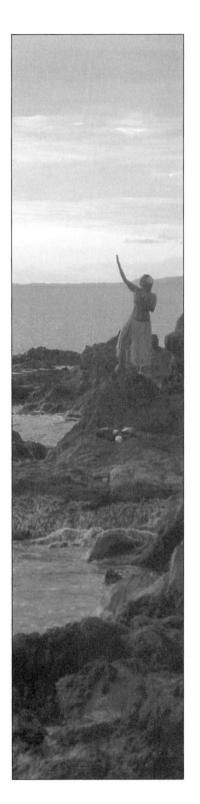

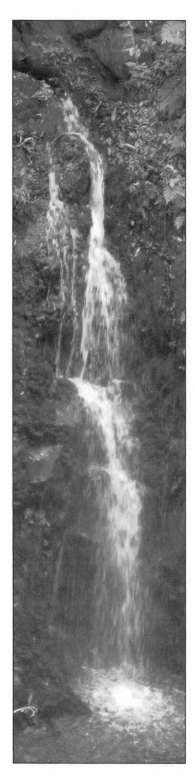

CONTENTS

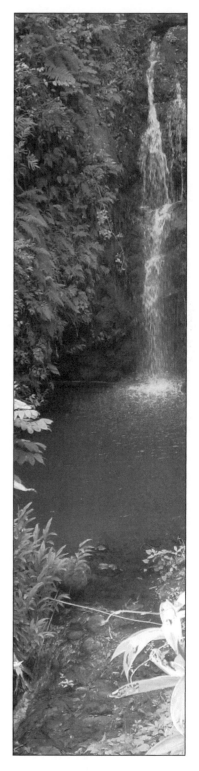

PREFACE
HOW TO USE THIS BOOK

This book presents acupressure points and techniques for treating a comprehensive range of emotional complaints and stress-related problems. The problems treated are organized alphabetically to make it easy for you to find a specific imbalance. Before turning to the chapter on a particular problem, however, we recommend that you at least read Chapters 1 and 3 to gain a knowledgeable foundation for treating yourself and for using acupressure safely and effectively.

Each chapter topic is self-contained, so you can skip around using the table of contents, the Quick Reference Guide on page 51, or the index. In each chapter you will find an introduction to the causes and issues related to the emotional complaint, a short story of how we applied acupressure for healing, positive affirmations, point descriptions with anatomical line drawings for determining the location and benefits, quick tips or miniroutines to use anywhere, and lastly, a self-care routine with step-by-step instructions for how to use the points.

Acupressure enables you to participate actively in your own healing. At the same time, however, you should continue to see your doctor or therapist for examinations, advice, and treatment. This book is not intended as a substitute for medical advice, but it can complement your medical care by enabling you to take a vital role in getting and staying well.

We hope that this book will lead you to a new dimension of well-being—not only to improve your health but to open the spirit within your heart and expand the awareness of your own healing energy. Simply using your hands to empower yourself—anytime, anywhere—is a tremendous blessing.

The reflections of water can symbolically portray the depth and flow of our emotions. The photographs of water throughout this book were taken with this in mind by Michael Reed Gach.

ABOUT THE AUTHORS

In the 1970s I (Michael Gach) studied Gestalt therapy and integrated its here-and-now techniques in my acupressure sessions with remarkable effectiveness. I discovered later that my unique way of guiding clients was similar to Focusing, a clinical approach for guiding clients into their inner awareness, formulated by Eugene Gendlin, PhD. As acupressure points are held, I coach a person to relax and breathe deeply to heighten their inner awareness. I have found that this process effectively releases unfinished emotional or traumatic experiences that have been stored within the body. As the acupressure points open, energy flows—awakening transformational healing experiences.

After twenty years of using acupressure for emotional balancing, I met Beth Henning in one of my acupressure trainings. Her written case studies assigned in the training had profound depth and vivid detail, demonstrating her understanding and skill in the emotional healing process. While cocreating this book with me, she has maintained a full-time acupressure practice combining breathwork, Reiki, and shamanism. Although we share many core beliefs and practices, we also incorporate different styles of healing methods. I believe our collaboration adds great depth to the scope and effectiveness of this book.

— *Michael Reed Gach, Dipl ABT, PhD*

I (Beth Henning) have been an alternative health clinician for twenty years, having studied with a variety of healers and spiritual teachers. My private practice consists of individuals who have exhausted mainstream health care or who cannot participate due to cost or personal preference.

Pain from a car accident in the late 1980s forced me to seek body-oriented therapies. All the valuable healings I had given others did not prepare me for handling my own debilitating chronic pain. As a single parent in private practice, I began a deep healing journey. During my recovery I studied, apprenticed, and cotaught with Michael Gach. Students found that our collaboration bridged many different psychological and spiritual aspects of natural healing. Acupressure changed my life and the direction of my private practice.

I continue to have incredible success teaching self-acupressure for home-care support. I have found no other natural healing method as powerful for balancing emotions and restoring health. I feel honored to share my experience and clinical knowledge as a partner on this inspiring project.

— *Beth Ann Henning, Dipl ABT*

GUIDELINES & PRECAUTIONS

Since the acupressure routines in this book are powerful techniques for emotional balancing, a strong release of feelings and memories can occur spontaneously. Thus, follow these guidelines to ensure your safety.

Psychotherapy

Be sure to see a counselor or psychotherapist for support if you have been severely traumatized or abused, emotionally or physically, and have the following recurring experiences:

- uncontrollable emotions, obsessions, or fantasies
- excessive anxiety, confusion, fear, depression, nightmares, or rage
- suicidal thoughts and tendencies
- chronic fatigue or emotional instability
- disorientation, dissociation, or difficulties coping with your life

We highly recommend that you work with a psychotherapist as a complement to the self-care techniques in this book. Such outside support can be essential. Combining acupressure's body-oriented therapy with psychotherapy results in increased effectiveness.

Regular Practice

Practice regularly, whether you are using acupressure to maintain your emotional health or to relieve a specific ailment. If you are using acupressure to relieve an ailment, continue using these same points even after you've obtained relief to prevent recurrence. If you cannot practice every day, treating yourself to acupressure two or three times a week can still be effective.

Medications

If you are taking medical or psychotropic medications, your system is at the mercy of these powerful drugs, which are controlling your metabolism. Setting limits is wise for maintaining stability. To be on the safe side, limit your acupressure sessions to ten minutes. If you feel stable, slowly increase the time by five minutes each week, working up to a full routine of approximately thirty minutes.

Both psychotropic medications and acupressure affect neurotransmitters, but acupressure has no negative side effects. Acupressure increases circulation, which can increase the absorption of a prescribed medication. Thus, after receiving acupressure, patients may feel overmedicated. Be sure to consult your doctor if you have any questions about your dosage. If your doctor recommends a smaller dosage, you are making progress in rebalancing your body's internal chemistry.

Acupressure Point Reference Book

All of the points in this book have numerous physical health benefits beyond what is listed here. If you are interested in learning more acupressure point applications for common complaints, refer to: *Acupressure's Potent Points* by Michael Reed Gach, PhD (New York: Bantam Books, 1991).

PART I:

FOUNDATIONS FOR EMOTIONAL HEALING

Today, mind/body research is confirming what ancient healing traditions have always known: that the body and the mind are a unity. There is no disease that isn't mental and emotional as well as physical.

— Christiane Northrup, MD
Women's Bodies, Women's Wisdom

1

ACUPRESSURE FOR EMOTIONAL WELL-BEING

WHAT IS ACUPRESSURE?

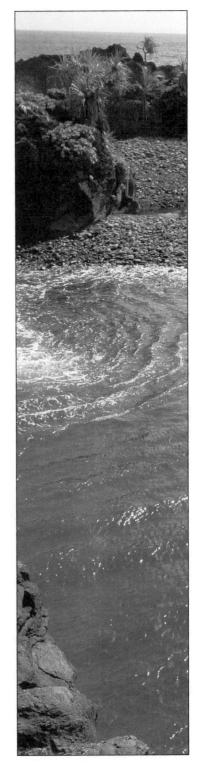

More than five thousand years ago the Chinese discovered that by applying pressure with their fingers and hands to specific points on the body, they could relieve pain. Through instinct, trial and error, and methodical observation, they identified hundreds of acupressure points that could be used to alleviate physical symptoms, benefit the healthy functioning of internal organs, and balance the emotions.

Acupressure stimulates the same points as acupuncture, but instead of needles, it uses the gentle but firm pressure of the hands to release muscular tension, promote the circulation of blood, and stimulate the body's natural self-curative abilities. Acupressure reaches to the core many of the emotional disorders and stress-related physical problems that typify our contemporary world. By freeing unresolved emotional experiences stored in the body, acupressure can alleviate a wide range of everyday aches and pains, allergies, poor circulation, sleeplessness, and other chronic complaints. It can even unveil the memory of a traumatic experience that caused an emotional wound.

For years Sally complained about being anxious and tense, which resulted in recurring headaches. As a store manager at age thirty-four, she was finding her emotional stress and physical complaints severely draining. She had chronic tension in her neck and a curvature in her upper back. Her relationship with her boyfriend was stressful and further exacerbated her pain. She felt overwhelmed; making decisions was especially difficult.

Sally took an acupressure class, where she learned points to relieve her pain at home. As she held her neck and the pressure points under the base of her skull with her eyes closed, she remembered a fight with a boy in second grade: he had pushed her back so abruptly that her neck was traumatized with whiplash. She recalled how her head filled with pressure as her teacher reprimanded her in front of the class. Since then she had suffered from anxiety attacks and head pain. Holding the acupressure points on her own neck enabled Sally to recall and reexperience the source of her trauma. She began seeing a psychotherapist and a bodyworker. One month after practicing self-acupressure twice a day, she reported that her neck tension, headaches, and anxiety had dissipated; she felt clearer, empowered, and more self-reliant.

Acupressure relaxes the tight muscles that result from an emotional trauma. A traumatic event causes the body to contract its muscles and harden, like protective armor, to shield the inner self. For instance, when something frightens you or someone uptight treats you abrasively, your neck and shoulders may tighten immediately in response. This tension prevents energy from circulating freely in your body. As a result, your body may overreact and shut down, causing various physical ailments and emotional imbalances. If you do not deal with these tensions and resulting afflictions, emotional problems may resurface. Most therapies address the cognitive and emotional aspects of trauma but do not get to the physiological component. Acupressure has an advantage over these therapies in that its techniques work directly with the body that has been affected by the trauma.

Emotional imbalances and the physical symptoms that accompany them are often the body's response to unresolved issues and events. A tension headache, for instance, may be caused by a conflict at work or an argument over homework with one's teenager. Someone who witnessed a fatal automobile accident may live with the memory of burning bodies and twisted metal in the form of recurring nightmares and insomnia; if left untreated they can continue for years. Divorce, even when it seems amicable, is a life-changing transition that can cause both emotional problems (like anxiety, worry, and moderate depression) and physical symptoms (such as stomachaches, ulcers, irritable bowel problems, and more).

Brenda, a forty-two-year-old computer programmer, went for an acupressure session because she had been suffering from insomnia and anxiety ever since her bitter divorce three years earlier. The divorce process was a series of traumatic, emotionally painful experiences. She felt drained and depressed, but she didn't have a history of depression, and she didn't think depression ran in her family. Her doctor prescribed Prozac for the depression and Xanax for her nervousness and fatigue. She tried biofeedback to help her relax, and cognitive-behavioral therapy to deal with her constant negative thoughts. She found that neither the medications nor the various other therapies she tried transformed her ongoing depressed state of mind. Her depression fluctuated between apathy and despair.

Finally, Brenda took a friend's advice and got in touch with Michael Gach. During the first sessions, they worked on her back, and in her abdomen. Michael showed her emotional balancing points on her upper neck and chest for the anxiety-related headaches, and upper back stretching exercises and ankle points for the insomnia. After using self-acupressure and breathing exercises daily for a month, Brenda felt more relaxed and self-reliant. Holding the points in her upper neck reduced the frequency and severity of her headaches. After three months of self-treatment her sleep improved, she had more energy, and a decrease in her anxiety. Acupressure released most of the tension that Brenda had accumulated and carried in the aftermath of her marital split, making emotional resolution possible. In addition, she gained a renewed connection with her body, restoring her vitality and touching her aliveness.

Our bodies are constantly making adjustments to accommodate the demands (some would say unnatural demands) of modern technology. People who work at their desks, typing away at a computer keyboard and straining their eyes to see the screen, are no strangers to headaches, tense shoulders, stiff neck, backaches, shallow breathing, and repetitive injuries like carpal tunnel syndrome.

Television, computers, and video games are also major causes of the obesity epidemic. Poor eating habits, stress in the workplace or at home, chronic muscular tension, lack of exercise, and bad posture contribute to lethargy, depression, and apathy. Acupressure can rebalance your body and enable you to cope with the demands of modern life.

FOUNDATIONS OF ACUPRESSURE & EMOTIONAL HEALING

Using this natural healing art has no side effects. Your hands are the only equipment you need. The art of acupressure utilizes the sensitivity of the human hand to release endorphins, your body's natural pain-relieving chemicals. These neurochemicals are released by your pituitary gland and get distributed through the cerebrospinal fluid into the bloodstream. Simply holding certain points with steady, firm pressure for a few minutes will release these pain-relief agents. We believe that endorphins also play an important role in cultivating both physical and emotional healing.

Tension and pain accumulate at acupressure points. As a point is held, muscular tension yields to finger pressure, enabling the fibers of the muscle to elongate and relax, blood to flow freely, and toxins to be released and eliminated. When blood and bioelectrical energy circulate properly, you have a greater sense of harmony, health, and well-being. As a result, your symptoms are alleviated, and your circulation is increased sufficiently to restore well-being.

Acupressure points have a high electrical conductivity at the surface of the skin. Holding a point allows life energy to flow through the body. Traditional Chinese medicine refers to this energy as *chi* (pronounced *chee*); in Japan it is known as *ki* (pronounced *key*). Western scientists have proven the existence of this energy by using microvolt meters, high-tech electrical devices that measure energy and electrical charge throughout the body.

Meridians are the energy pathways that connect acupressure points to one another and to the internal organs. Just as blood vessels nourish the body physically, meridians circulate healing energy to all systems of the body. There are twelve bilateral meridians that run along both sides of the body and relate to specific organs, and eight extraordinary vessels.

These pathways are a master communication system of universal life energy, connecting the organs with all sensory experiences.* An acupressure point in one part of the body can send a healing message to other parts of the body through the meridians. Applying pressure on certain points triggers the flow of energy through the meridian pathway. We call these *trigger points* because they are at a distance from the area they benefit.

The *limbic system,* a group of structures in the forebrain, has been called the center of our emotions. The limbic system requires energy to flow through the meridians to function properly, but stress and emotional disturbances inhibit the circulation of energy. The resulting tensions accumulate at acupressure points. As tension from stress builds or becomes chronic, blood circulation decreases, inhibiting body functions. Tightness in the chest can make breathing difficult. Using acupressure points on the chest can free breathing, reduce chest pain, and relieve depression. The balancing point on the center of the breastbone, for instance, is good for relieving dizziness and chest constriction, benefiting the cardiovascular system and calming the emotions.

In this book, you will find acupressure points used for a variety of emotional problems, many of which present themselves as physical symptoms. For instance, as you hold points underneath your skull to relieve a headache or insomnia, an insight may come that shifts your state of mind and thereby alleviates your anxiety. As you continue to open your body's energy by using acupressure, greater health, mental clarity, and an expanded awareness will occur, dissolving conflicts between mind and body.

---

*Harriet Beinfield, LAc, and Efrem Korngold, LAc, OMD, *Between Heaven and Earth: A Guide to Chinese Medicine* (New York: Ballantine, 1991).

HOW TO FIND A POINT

Names & Reference Numbers

You can locate acupressure points by using nearby anatomical landmarks, especially bony or muscular indicators. Acupressure points located underneath muscles, ligaments, or tendons feel like cords, bands, or knots of tension. Points located near a bone are found in the indentations of the bone or in the hollow created between bones.

Each of the 365 traditional acupressure points has a poetic name based on a Chinese character. The imagery of its name offers insight into its benefits or location. For instance, the point named Hidden Clarity is good for clearing the mind and emotions. Shoulder's Corner refers to the location of that point.

Some point names, such as Sea of Tranquility, provide insight into how that point can support your emotional healing process. Many of the healing visualizations and meditations in this book use points with names referring to their healing benefits. Point names can be used to create positive affirmations and amplify the benefits. For example, hold the Letting Go points on your upper, outer chest with your fingertips. Breathe deeply. Imagine yourself letting go of your frustration and tension. As you hold and breathe into these points, place your attention on your fingertips. Say to yourself, "I am letting go of my negative thoughts, anger, and resentment."

Each acupressure point also has an identification number to indicate its placement on the body. These point location numbers, such as CV 17 or B 10, are based on a standard referencing system used by professional acupressurists and acupuncturists. You can find what these abbreviations refer to by looking in the Glossary. You do not need to know or remember any of these numbers to practice the emotional healing techniques in this book.

How to Apply Pressure

The amount of pressure to apply depends on your body's state of health and fitness. The more developed your muscles are, the more pressure you should apply. If you feel pain, gradually decrease the pressure until you find a balance between pain and pleasure. The pressure should be firm enough to "hurt good." If a point is sore or painful, hold it lightly for a few minutes, and the pain will diminish.

The middle finger, the longest and strongest, is best suited for emotional healing. A major meridian travels through it. Use your middle finger to apply pressure, with your index and ring fingers on either side for support. The next time someone points their middle finger upward at you, hopefully they are sending healing energy your way.

The thumb is strong and excellent for applying pressure on areas of large muscle mass. Avoid using your thumb excessively on an area that is sensitive. If you need more pressure but your hand hurts when you apply finger pressure, use your knuckles, fists, or some other tool, like a tennis or golf ball. You can obtain massage tools at health food stores as well.

Sometimes when you hold a point, you'll feel pain in another part of your body. This *referred pain* is caused when a blocked area in one part of the body causes symptoms in another. Often the pain moves to another area because of a blockage in the meridian pathway.

Richard, a forty-three-year-old furniture sales-man, often felt emotionally frustrated; his chronic hip, shoulder, and neck tension was caused by a blockage in his Gall Bladder meridian. His referred pain followed the meridian pathway down the outside of his leg. We will show you how to use local and distal points that work with the meridians to send healing energy to a blocked area.

Acupressure is most effective when the points are held steadily with direct finger pressure at a 90-degree angle from the surface of the skin. The correct pressure is applied slowly, directed toward the center of the body. Applying pressure in this way avoids pulling the skin. To achieve a deeper, longer-lasting healing response, release the finger pressure gradually, and end with about twenty seconds of light touch.

When you hold a point in a conscious way for at least three minutes while you breathe slowly and deeply, you may feel a pulsation at that point. This pulsation is a good sign—it means your circulation has increased, and tension and pain may diminish. Pay attention to the type of pulsation you feel. If it's throbbing or very faint, hold the point until the rhythm becomes more balanced and smooth. If you do not feel a pulsation, you may notice other signs of release, like temperature increase, yawning, eyes fluttering, or a release of muscle tightness.

For emotional healing, we encourage you to hold the points for a couple of minutes at a time. At first your hands may tire or the muscles of your arms may ache, but after several months of daily practice, your hand muscles will strengthen. To relieve fatigue in your hands, rotate your wrists, gently shake your hands out, and take a few deep breaths. Return to the point and apply pressure gradually.

Once you have located the point and your fingers are comfortably positioned, gradually lean your body weight toward the point to apply pressure. This will enable you to apply firm pressure without strain. When you use the muscles only of your arms and hands to apply pressure, you may tend to go too fast into a point, which can be unnecessarily painful.

Each person's body and each area of the body requires a different amount of pressure. The calves, the face, and the genital and abdominal areas are more sensitive and thus need lighter pressure. Muscular areas of the body, such as the back, buttocks, and shoulders, usually need deeper, firmer pressure. You may find that each point feels somewhat different when you press it; some points may feel sore or ache, while others may be tense or feel good.

Benefits of Self-Care

Self-care has the following benefits:

- **Accessibility to Practice Anytime, Anywhere:** You do not need any special tools or have to make advance appointments. You can practice in your office or in the comfort of your home, whenever you want.

- **Individualized Treatment Touch:** While pressing your own points, you can easily determine how much pressure feels right to you. If it's too hard, you will immediately reduce the pressure. You can also try applying pressure at different angles, feeling which approach is most beneficial.

- **Self-Reliance:** These techniques are empowering; you do not have to depend on anyone else for them. The independence you gain by practicing self-care will heighten your morale and outlook.

- **Unlimited Cost-Free Treatments:** When you know how to practice acupressure on yourself, no costs are involved.

- **Connection with Your Body:** Self-care cultivates an inner healing relationship with yourself that is nurturing and grounding. This connection fosters trust and healing and increases your awareness of your body's unique expressions and wisdom.

ACUPRESSURE PRECAUTIONS

Acupressure's healing touch is safe to do on yourself and others as long as you pay attention to some basic commonsense precautions.

Patients with life-threatening diseases and serious medical problems should always consult their doctor before receiving acupressure. Avoid the abdominal area if you have intestinal cancer, tuberculosis, a serious cardiac condition, or leukemia.

Avoid the abdominal area during pregnancy. Be more gentle and careful when applying acupressure to a pregnant woman.

Apply finger pressure gradually to enable the tissue layers to respond in a healing manner. Never press into the body abruptly. If an area hurts excessively when you apply pressure, use a light touch instead.

Use a lighter, more sensitive touch in the lymph areas, such as the throat, groin, below the ears, and the outer breast near the armpits.

Do not press directly on a serious burn until it has healed.

Ulcerous conditions and infections should receive medical care.

Do not work directly on a recently formed scar or tumor. During the first month after an injury or operation, do not apply pressure directly onto the affected site.

Avoid practicing self-acupressure under the influence of alcohol or drugs.

Acupressure Preparation Guidelines

To prepare for an acupressure session, follow these guidelines.

Eat lightly or not at all before practicing acupressure; avoid having a full stomach prior to a session. Wait two or three hours after eating a heavy meal and at least an hour after a light meal. Practicing a complete acupressure routine when your stomach is full can inhibit the flow of blood and may cause nausea (although simply pressing one or two points can be perfectly safe).

Get enough sleep to feel fully rested.

Wear extra clothing and keep warm during and after an acupressure session to prevent chills. During acupressure your body's vital energies are concentrating inward to maximize healing; thus your body may produce less heat.

Wear comfortable clothing. Tight collars, belts, pants, or shoes can obstruct circulation. We recommend wearing natural fibers that breathe, such as cotton and wool. Rayon is also a good choice.

Keep your fingernails trimmed fairly short to prevent discomfort when applying pressure.

Practice Guidelines

During the acupressure session, follow these guidelines to obtain the full emotional healing benefits.

Find a comfortable, private environment where you can deeply relax. Choose a comfortable position, either sitting or lying down. As you press points in different areas, position your body to relax completely.

Limit your session to an hour. At first, your hands may ache while you hold a point for several minutes. Gradually work up to holding points longer, but do not hold any one point longer than ten minutes. Working on any single area of the body, such as the abdomen or face, for longer than twenty minutes can be excessive and cause an imbalance. The effects of acupressure can be quite strong. If you work too long, too much energy is released, and complications, such as nausea and headaches, can occur. If you feel lightheaded after a session, use caution and do not drive until you feel stable and alert.

Follow-Up Guidelines

After the session, follow these guidelines.

- **Have a trustworthy friend or counsel available for support,** and call this person if you feel unstable.

- **Observe the dietary considerations** in Chapter 26.

  Eat well, in moderation. Get enough protein to feel stable.

  Avoid sweets. Sugars, when eaten excessively, can cause many types of emotional instability. (See Chapter 21.)

  Avoid iced drinks. Extreme cold can weaken your system and counteract the benefits of acupressure. After an acupressure session, a cup of hot herbal tea would be good, followed by a nap for deep relaxation.

- **Deeply relax** after an acupressure session to get the most healing benefits and integrate the experience.

2

SPIRIT OF THE EMOTIONS

To me, all feelings are part of the wonderful, ever-changing sensation of being alive. If we love the different feelings, they become so many rainbow colors of life.

— Shakti Gawain
Living in the Light

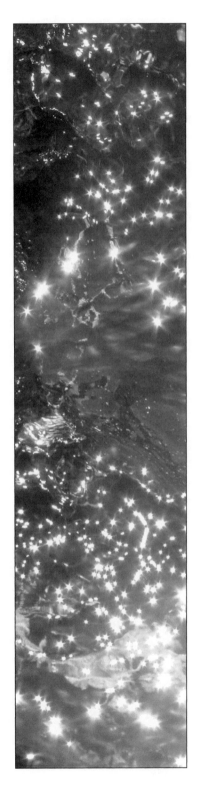

O ur most powerful spiritual experiences are rooted in the body. The life energy flowing through your body's points and meridians is the essence of your spirit—the source of your enthusiasm, vitality, and inner being. Emotional pain inhibits this energy from flowing. Tension from an emotional wound constricts life energy, much as a muscle contracts after an injury.

In children energy flows freely, creating their exuberant nature. Like a new, delicate seedling, however, a child's spirit is easily trampled; since their emotions are so open, children are vulnerable to being hurt. Hearing their parents raise their voices even at each other can be traumatic for children, let alone having their parents vent directly at them.

Many adult emotional issues stem from traumatic childhood events. Healing the inner child that we carry inside us as adults is fundamental for emotional healing; thus we highly recommend that you practice the Inner Child Healing Journey at the end of this chapter.

According to Chinese medicine, the heart not only propels blood but also governs your spirit. Your ability to open to love is called *shen,* the spirit of the heart. When you have *shen,* your body is in balance and harmony; you are able to make wise, life-enhancing choices. Acupressure, when practiced with deep breathing, stretching, and proper nutrition, helps you achieve *shen*.

Lorraine was a happy, spontaneous, and adventurous child who loved to play, dance, and perform for her parents and siblings. People of all ages were drawn to her zest for life and her carefree spirit. Unfortunately, Lorraine's older brother made her life miserable with his constant bullying and abuse. For Lorraine, his so-called playing—tricking, trapping, and teasing her to the point of tears—was a form of torture that dampened her spirit, traumatizing the young girl. An astute adult or child therapist would have recognized his behavior for what it was: emotional and verbal abuse. His manipulative nature and dominance, and her parents' inability to protect her from him, also affected her self-image. Anxiety, self-doubt, and ultimately, depression—in place of spiritedness and creativity—became the hallmarks of Lorraine's childhood and adolescence.

As she grew into adulthood, Lorraine's depression worsened, affecting her relationships and her ability to express herself. Her spirit was wounded. The unexpressed anger, resentment, and unresolved trauma from her years of emotional abuse led to physical problems such as sluggishness, breathing difficulties, insomnia, and nightmares. Lorraine found relief in yoga classes and bodywork. Acupressure classes further facilitated her ability to help herself. After several months she was feeling more in tune with her body, was sleeping better, and felt more at peace with herself.

The Spiritual Nature of the Emotions

Your emotions are your body's natural responses to your life experiences. They are an intimate communication system, expressing your inner reality from moment to moment. Emotional tension can inhibit circulation, cause fatigue, and disrupt focus and concentration. You know what muscle tension and stiffness feel like and how stress affects your perceptions and moods. Over time, emotionally distressful experiences hamper your ability to be fully responsive and in the moment.

How many times have you heard that your face can be read as easily as a book? Joy, anger, frustration, sadness—laugh lines, frown lines, worry lines—change the shape and characteristics of your face. Similarly, negative feelings such as resentment, chronic fear, self-doubt, and worry consume your vitality and have a powerful and damaging effect on your body's internal systems.

You cannot be fully responsive and spiritually vital if past emotional wounds remain unhealed and keep you from feeling your body. You cannot trust your intuition, make wise decisions, or take care of yourself if your emotional responses are restrained. Cultivating body awareness and learning to trust your feelings through acupressure will enable you to fully embrace your spirituality.

Trust & Faith

Spiritual growth requires trust and faith. Trusting your perceptions enables you to be independent, and fully experience your spirituality—to grasp how everything in life is interconnected. If you do not care for yourself or listen to and trust your own feelings, you can easily become dependent on others. If you do not trust the messages of your body due to a past traumatic experience, your body becomes numb and shuts off. A wounded heart has a limited capacity to trust and be open to infinite possibilities. Emotional numbness can create codependent relationships; dependency occurs when you lack self-esteem or harbor a poor body image.

Childhood traumatic events, which are so common, at any young age—jeopardize trust and faith—thus eclipsing the exuberant wonder of the child's spirit. The Inner Child Healing Journey at the end of this chapter can guide you to reconnect with your inner child, restoring the trust and faith you once had for renewing your spirit. The following story, like so many of the stories in this book, shows how emotional problems in adult life stem from childhood traumas and dependent relationships.

Judy, a single woman in her mid-forties, had a consistent pattern of codependent love relationships. Her pattern is a familiar one for many women who have been overwhelmed by life's circumstances and who lose themselves trying to meet the needs of their partners. Codependency is also known as "relationship addiction," because people with codependency usually get themselves into relationships that are one-sided, emotionally destructive, and often physically abusive. How did Judy, a social worker who was held in high regard by her colleagues, develop such low self-esteem and harbor a dangerously poor body image? Why had she become so disconnected from herself and her feelings?

Judy was emotionally hurt as a child. Her parents fought bitterly and divorced when she was seven. Both parents tried to lure her to their side with sugarcoated promises, while bitterly blaming each other. The guilt caused by her parents' traumatic arguments caused an unresolved emotional wound in Judy that cut her off from trusting and coping with the world of intimacy as an adult woman. She was attracted to unhealthy, emotionally abusive, and dependent relationships. Each romantic attraction triggered the child within her, longing for a stable relationship she could rely on. Whenever she fell in love, she would become overwhelmed and lose herself trying to meet the needs of her partner.

In counseling, Judy began to explore how she could change the negative relationships in her life. In her counseling sessions, she became familiar with the syndrome of codependency. As she talked about her past, she noticed over and over again how her body had absorbed the stresses and traumas from her childhood abuses. Her counselor recommended a massage therapist who practiced acupressure therapy. Acupressure opened Judy to feelings that she had blocked off for over thirty years. She felt as if her emotions were being squeezed out of her like a sponge. As her points were pressed, distressful issues related to her poor self-image and her feelings of self-doubt and inadequacy were released.

As Judy's traumatic experiences surfaced and she shed the pain within her heart, she regained her self-esteem through healing touch. Her acupressure massage therapist focused on emotional healing points in between the shoulder blades, where she had knots of tension. She also learned self-acupressure and practiced several times per day. Judy used St 13 (on the chest below the collarbone) and CV 6 (two inches below the navel). After many months of self-treatment, she rejoiced, "I've rediscovered my body and embrace my feelings as a cherished friend. I'm amazed; just a few months ago this same body felt rotten and insecure. I feel alive again." Judy's renewed spirit transformed her life; one year later she had a healthy, stable, intimate relationship.

The Legacy of Painful Memories

Negative emotional patterns can be passed from parent to child, but we still have much to learn about the linkage between genes and vulnerability to mood disorders. Although the heredity factors aren't conclusive, the transference of trauma and emotional hardships from generation to generation is noticeable.

Your parents' past traumatic experiences and the tension held within their bodies affected how they treated you as a child. If as children they experienced a short temper, irritability, scolding, and blame from their own parents, they most likely treated you and your siblings the same way. You can break this negative cycle by becoming aware of similar patterns in your own relationships. When you sense your irritability or impatience growing, hold your acupressure points while breathing deeply to foster more responsiveness to your feelings instead of being enslaved by them.

Your life reflects what you believe and can accept. Avoiding painful feelings and memories perpetuates personal suffering, but when you dwell on your emotional pain and suffering, you cultivate misery in your life. Is the purpose of your life to carry past hurts and oppressive memories?

Buried memories can be hard to recall if the experience was painful. Time has a way of fading perceptions, especially of traumatic experiences that were scary or hurtful. As you work with the self-care routines in this book and your memories surface, remember that emotional pain is an expression of real traumatic or painful experiences. We encourage you to unveil hidden memories; these recollections can be pivotal for reawakening your spirit.

Transforming Emotional Pain

Holding acupressure points can relieve emotional pain and be a catalyst for a profound spiritual realization. Memories, emotions, and spiritual insights are all amplified as acupressure opens the body's vital life energy.

You cannot feel joy when your heart is filled with pain. Behind your emotional pain are truths your body has registered from the past; without releasing that pain, you cannot experience the depths of pleasure.

Feelings of euphoria are common after an acupressure session in which emotional pain has been expressed and released. An emotional charge such as crying can release a tremendous amount of energy throughout the body. Tears can come to your eyes whether you are extremely happy or in pain. (Childbirth is an example of how the greatest pain can become the greatest pleasure.) Pain and pleasure produce similar neurochemical reactions. Acupressure activates endorphins, the neurochemicals that can give you a natural high.

Service to Others

Serving others consciously can fulfill your life's purpose as long as you maintain your own sense of self. Giving unconditionally of yourself releases pent-up pain and heightens your self-esteem and spirit; it also strengthens your immune system and reduces your risk of heart attacks and other debilitating illnesses.

Expressing your feelings, and your faith in the oneness of life by choosing to serve others will reduce your emotional stress. When your devotion to other fulfills your life's purpose and connects you with your higher self, your emotional pain eases. Serving others and being loving to yourself will open your heart to being healed.

VISUALIZATIONS FOR YOUR SPIRIT

Emotion is the chief source of all becoming conscious. There can be no transforming of darkness into light and of apathy into movement without emotion.

— C. G. Jung

The following visualizations can cultivate your spiritual development. The Third Eye point (GV 24.5) and the Hundred Meeting point (GV 20) are the most powerful acupressure points for clearing your mind and developing your spirituality. By lightly touching GV 24.5 with GV 20, you can enhance your inner awareness, intuition, emotional stability, and spiritual connection.

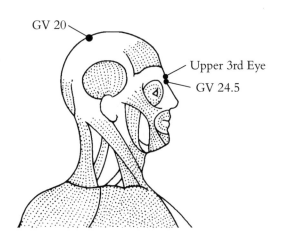

There are two different Third Eye point locations. The lower Third Eye point (GV 24.5) is located in the indentation where the bridge of the nose meets the forehead. The upper is located one thumb-width above where your eyebrows meet. Most people find that one of these points is more sensitive than the other. To find out which point is more beneficial for you, first lightly touch the lower point, between your eyebrows, and close your eyes. Experience the sensitivity of touching this point, then slowly release the contact. Next, gently hold the upper point, in the center of your forehead, and close your eyes again. Decide which point gave you a more powerful experience. Both of these points connect with the pituitary gland and have the same benefits.

The Hundred Meeting point (GV 20) is located on the crown of the head in an indentation or "soft spot" between the cranial bones. Find the point by following an imaginary line from the backs of your ears up to the top of your head. Holding this point improves mental concentration and memory and heightens spiritual awareness.

The following visualization on the Third Eye point (GV 24.5) and the Hundred Meeting point (GV 20) provides many healing benefits, including stress reduction, mental clarity, and greater spiritual awareness. Concentrating on the center of your forehead while lightly holding these powerful points also balances the emotions and can replace negative thinking with positive beliefs. Within a few weeks of daily visualization, you may notice an increase in your intuition—your ability to envision and manifest your dreams.

You may want to record these two visualizations by slowly reading them aloud into a tape recorder; then play this audio recording and follow the guided instructions.

Third Eye Visualization

Find a quiet space where you can meditate for three to five minutes twice a day. Close your eyes, and sit in a comfortable position with your spine straight. Place your middle fingertip lightly on the Third Eye point (GV 24.5), and hold it throughout this meditation. Focus your attention between your eyebrows, straighten your spine, and begin to breathe deeply…

Become aware of every part of your body while you breathe into the Third Eye point. As you inhale, imagine that the incoming air is streaming through the center of your forehead… Let this air filter through your whole body as you exhale smoothly and slowly… Gently gaze inward with your eyes closed, raising your eyebrows up, and roll your eyes also upward and inward as you put your concentration on your Third Eye point… Imagine

pleasurable warmth in the center of your forehead… Continue to breathe deeply as you welcome this warm healing energy coming through you…

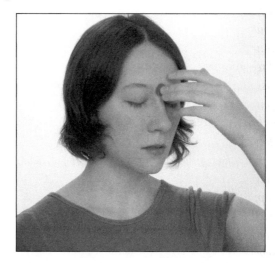

Now use your other hand to hold the Hundred Meeting point at the crown of your head, and imagine air going through it like the spout of a whale or dolphin… As you breathe deeply, visualize a stream of air rushing through the dolphin hole on the top of your head… Suck the air in through your spout for another minute…

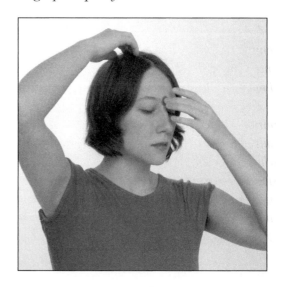

Make your inhalation swift and deep... At the top of the inhalation, hold your breath for a few seconds to assimilate the oxygen... Exhale slowly and smoothly, letting healing energy move throughout your body... Now bring your hands down to rest into your lap, palms facing up. Keep your focus on the depth of each breath for the next three minutes... With each long, slow, deep breath, visualize yourself pumping healing energy into your body, fortifying your body's cells... Continue to breathe deeply for a couple more minutes as you notice what you discover...

Focus on bringing life energy from the earth into your feet... Feel the gravitational force of the earth supporting your body. Take a few minutes to come back from this meditation. Rotate your hands on your wrists, and rotate your feet on your ankles several times. Stretch your arms and legs as you take some deep breaths and slowly open your eyes.

Heightening Awareness Visualization

Practice the following guided imagery exercise in front of a mirror.

Sit in a comfortable chair, and let your entire body relax completely... During this exercise stay connected to your breath. To deepen your experience, you will be reminded to breathe deeply throughout this visualization.

As you take deep breaths, look at yourself in the mirror... Come closer to the mirror, and notice details of how you look... Breathe deeply and notice what comes up as you explore your facial expressions... As you look into the mirror, notice what your image is conveying... Take some deep breaths into your heart as you come closer to notice what expressions are in your eyes... What is your posture saying to you? Continue breathing deeply... exploring your movements, and feelings.

Now use all your fingertips to firmly hold Heavenly Pillar on the back of your neck on both sides (B 10). Without saying any words, imagine your image can speak to you. Ask the image to give you advice about a troublesome or traumatic experience. Continue to breathe deeply as you explore your feelings and facial expressions . . .

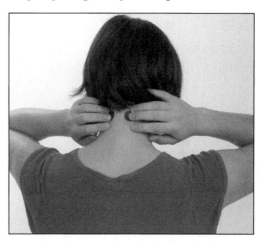

Now close your eyes and explore a part of your body that feels tight or blocked. Check out your jaws, shoulders, and stomach... Notice what part of your body aches, hurts, or feels tired... Take a deep breath into one of these areas... Have the courage to focus on how it feels...

Place your fingers on the place where you feel most uncomfortable or have the most tension. Breathe right into that spot... Adjust the location and depth of the pressure to make direct contact. Bring all your attention to that spot, and ask yourself how it feels or what it looks like... Continue to breathe into it as you ask yourself, "What caused this problem?" Breathe deeply, and listen for the answer...

When an answer comes or your tension subsides, slowly release the pressure, holding the area lightly... then take another deep breath, coming off slowly as your hands come down into your lap—letting yourself completely relax.

When you feel, you gain awareness.
Through this increased spiritual awareness,
You will have the focus to deal with a problem.

SPIRITUAL PRACTICES FOR
TRANSFORMING THE EMOTIONS

Emotions can be used as allies for your spiritual growth. In this section, we will explore how several different emotions can be used constructively for spiritual development and transformation.

Transforming Fear

The spirit of fear arises to guide you in knowing and trusting your limits. When you have gone beyond your comfort zone or are confronted with the unknown, fear immediately surfaces to let you know what is safe for you. Fear is almost always a reaction to your body's perception of a limit, danger, or threat. Instead of avoiding fear, use the opportunity it presents to face challenges for going deeper within your soul. Normally people close their senses to protect themselves from what is frightening. Fear can open your senses to your spiritual growth and empowerment if you listen to what the spirit of fear is trying to teach you. Most people discover that transformation occurs when they have faced their fears and have come out on the other side.

Acupressure self-care can support you to embrace your fears in a courageous way to fuel your spirit. When you are afraid, holding K 27 (Elegant Mansion) supports you to breathe deeply instead of breathing shallowly and shutting down. To find K 27, place your fingertips on your chest and firmly press into the inden-

tations directly below the protrusions of the collarbone. Hold this point while taking long, deep, slow breaths for two to three minutes.

Whenever you are afraid, remember to breathe slowly and deeply. Breathing shallowly during scary times doesn't supply enough oxygen to give you the essential energy you need to respond, so let your fear be a signal to take deep breaths. By breathing deeply into your fear, you can empower yourself, increase your awareness, and receive the wise messages fear presents for spiritual guidance. Normally, fear shuts down the breath. But, by breathing deeply, you can transform

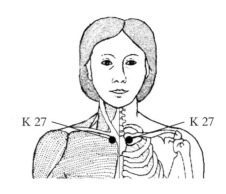

K 27   K 27

fear into a sense of awe, awakening a full range of genuine responses.

Expressing your fear can cultivate intimacy by opening yourself and your partner to the unknown. Intimacy can make you feel vulnerable at first. Breathing slowly and deeply into whatever is scary can enable you to share and express your inner self—opening a sense of wonder, emotional sensitivity, and insight.

According to traditional Chinese medicine, the urinary bladder and kidney meridians govern not only fear but also the water element. Fear, like water, is a vast ocean containing depths of the unknown. Water flows, moistens, nourishes, and sustains life. Like water, fear can awaken your spirit and deepen your emotions. Just as you can drown in excessive water, you can drown in or be overwhelmed by a flood of fears. Instead of being overwhelmed by your fears, explore them by breathing deeply, expanding your scope of awareness. Use fear's lesson as a guide to heighten your awareness and enrich your spirit through the following practice.

Spiritual Practices for Transforming Fear

Sit up on the edge of your chair for this routine for cultivating an alliance with fear—developing the spirit of guidance.

Rub B 23 & B 47 (Sea of Vitality): Briskly rub these points in your lower back with the backs of your hands for one minute. Use friction to create heat; warming your lower back benefits your kidneys, the organ that governs fear. Rubbing your lower back vigorously for one minute, one to five times daily, can strengthen your kidneys, endowing you with the courage to face your fears. Finish by placing your hands comfortably in your lap and resting for one minute.

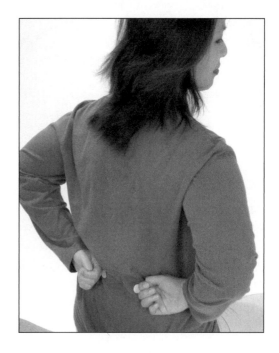

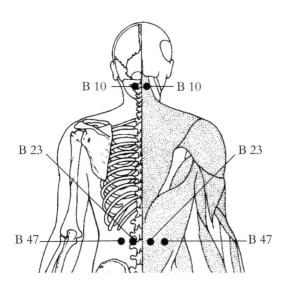

Hold K 27 (Elegant Mansion): Place your fingertips on your chest and firmly press K 27 (in the indentations directly below the protrusions of the collarbone).

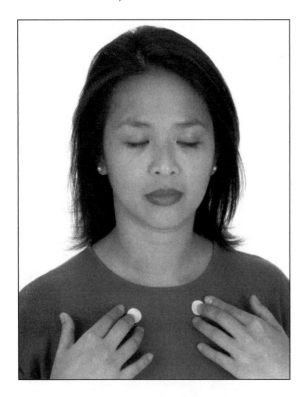

Take slow, deep breaths as you firmly hold these spiritually uplifting points for one minute. Close your eyes and focus your concentration on taking long, deep breaths into these points for two minutes; this clears your chest and spirit.

Meditate on breathing deeply into any fears, scary dreams, or catastrophic fantasies. As you breathe slowly and deeply, notice what feelings, images, and thoughts are connected to your fear, to gain an awareness of what your spirit is trying to teach you.

Transforming Anger

The purpose of emotions, regardless of what they are, is to help us feel and participate fully in our own lives. To become aware of our inner guidance system, we must learn to trust our emotions.

— Christiane Northrup, MD
Women's Bodies, Women's Wisdom

Most people associate anger with its negative attributes: unresolved resentment, outrage, and hostility. Repressed anger can cause numbness, apathy, and depression, inhibiting your desire to strive toward your highest dreams. Excessive anger turns to rage and even fury. When mixed with jealousy and boundary issues, anger can result in violence. But through deep breathing, determination, and positive thinking, you can learn to transform anger into an empowering, creative force that supports your life's purpose.

When your willpower is directed toward healthy personal goals, this motivating force can boost your spirit and help you create what you want in your life. As we'll see in Chapter 7, anger thoughtfully expressed and balanced through a program of self-acupressure, exercise, and diet, produces the energy to initiate change. Channeled in a creative direction, the spirit of anger's willful force can fuel your aspirations and visions.

By teaching you to channel anger creatively, acupressure can enable you to grasp some of the greatest spiritual teachings. Anger is a powerful driving force for expressing your innermost needs and increasing your spiritual awareness. Balanced anger enables you to stand up for yourself. Next time you feel agitated or irritable, instead of repressing or venting your anger inappropriately, hold your middle finger firmly to stimulate the emotional balancing energies of the Pericardium meridian. Taking several slow, full breaths as you hold your middle finger can direct this assertive force within you to articulate what you need.

Several months ago Nathan, an acupressure student, had a revealing insight about his anger. While receiving acupressure from a fellow student, Nathan realized that his ordinary shoulder and neck tension was reflecting not only his frustration about his work but also his anger and resentment for the way he was being treated there. Even when he thought everything was fine, acupressure uncovered perceptions and emotions that he was then able to address. Behind his mask of happiness, several anger issues were stored within his mid- to upper back region, shoulders, and neck. By expressing his anger, Nathan was able to be assertive, stand up for himself, and reclaim his aliveness. To sustain the results, he gave himself daily acupressure using the following emotional balancing points on the chest, shoulders, and neck.

Spiritual Practices for Transforming Anger

Sit up comfortably in a chair and begin breathing deeply to hold the following points for balancing anger:

Press B 10 (Heavenly Pillar, located on the back of your upper neck one finger-width below your skull and one finger-width out from the center of the spine on both sides): Breathe deeply while you hold B 10 on both sides of the neck. To make sure you are on these points, curve your fingers and place all of your fingertips on the thick ropy muscles on the back of your neck. Apply firm pressure on these muscles as you move your head up and down for one minute. Inhale as you raise your head up slowly and gently back—exhale as you let your head come forward. Maintain firm pressure as you repeat this movement five more times while breathing deeply. Heavenly Pillar is a spiritual point for heightening self-expression and the relationship between mind and body.

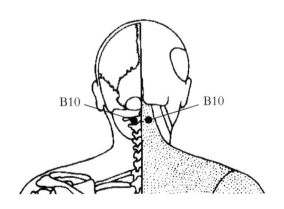

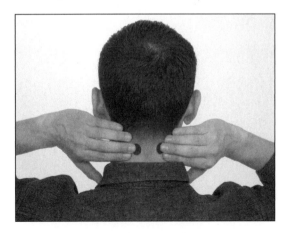

Press CV 17 (Sea of Tranquility, located on the center of the breastbone, four finger-widths up from the bone's base): Bring the palms of your hands together at the center of your chest.

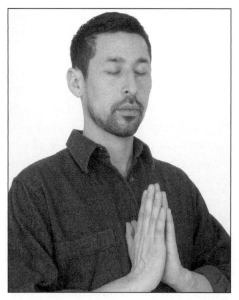

Use the back knuckles of your thumbs to press CV 17 (in the small indentation of your breastbone). Close your eyes, and breathe slowly and deeply into your heart for two minutes to calm yourself.

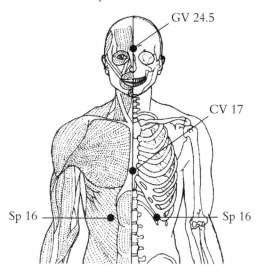

Transforming Worry & Self-Doubt

If you are worried about a problem in the future, imagine yourself in the fearful situation. Then imagine that you are coping with it, or even enjoying it.

— Emrika Padus
The Complete Guide to Your Emotions and Your Health

Worrying and overthinking suppress your energy system and many body functions: your breathing gets shallow, your stomach becomes acidic, and your blood sugar levels fluctuate. In addition, chronic worry leads to eating disorders, especially sugar cravings. Over time these metabolic imbalances can cause debilitating conditions such as chronic fatigue syndrome, immune system deficiencies, and fibromyalgia. When you worry, you lose touch with the present moment. How can you be in touch with your spirit if you are fatigued, unable to cope with the stresses of the day, and preoccupied with myriad physical problems?

Trust is the basis for emotional and spiritual growth. Worry strangles your spirit and depletes your vital energy. Acupressure, deep breathing exercises, and practicing the techniques of positive thinking are effective measures for trusting yourself and counteracting worry's harmful influences.

Spiritual Practices for Transforming Worry

Hold Sp 16 (Abdominal Sorrow, at the base of the ribcage): Certain points become blocked when you worry excessively. For instance, worry can create abdominal tension in the diaphragm. To release the tension in these points, interlace your fingers with the palms of your hands on your stomach area. With the tips of your thumbs together, place the base of your thumbs against the base of your ribcage.

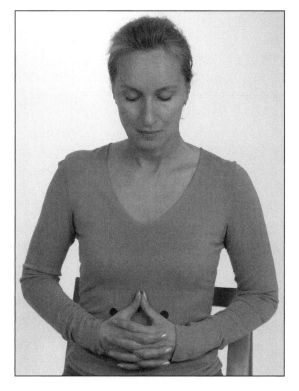

Connect with Sp 16 gently for two minutes as you focus on taking slow, deep breaths. Holding this point can reinforce a positive sense of self and cultivate your spirit.

Third Eye Meditation on Gratitude:
The following meditation counteracts worry by focusing on gratitude.

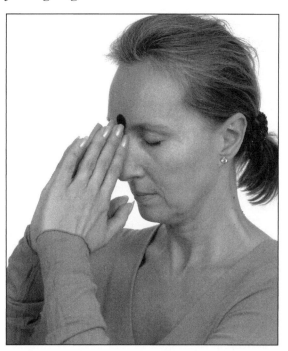

Sit up straight, close your eyes, and begin long, slow, deep breathing. For the next three minutes, focus on what you have to be grateful for… Place your middle fingertip gently on the Third Eye point (GV 24.5, in the indentation between your eyebrows). Imagine you are free of worry, self-doubt, and emotional pain. Holding the Third Eye point fortifies the pituitary gland, which activates the spirit, counteracts worry, and can transform guilt. Return to deep breathing and focusing on what you have to be grateful for as you slowly release your hands onto your lap. Rest for one minute with your eyes closed, taking deep breaths, to discover the benefits.

Transforming Grief & Sadness

When you lose someone you love, grieving releases your sadness, allowing you to let go of emotional attachment and pain. It also enables you to let go of your expectations and disappointments. Grieving is an emotional purification; crying opens the breath, allows you to let go, and renews your spirit. Holding on to your emotions stifles your spirit. When you are attached to what you love with expectation, you limit the flow of what is possible in life. Clutching to what you are accustomed to, expect, or desire blocks your connection with the infinite.

Grieving is a two-step process: feeling the grief, then healing it. Acupressure points are used to help you authentically feel a loss and the myriad emotions that accompany it. Once you have had adequate time to be with the hurt and have an outlet for expressing the emotional pain, acupressure can aid in the healing process.

Holding on to grief and sadness can create a wide range of problems in your chest and upper back. Heartaches, anguish, and depression constrict the chest muscles and commonly create knots between the shoulder blades. According to traditional Chinese medicine, this tension binds the respiratory apparatus, inhibits deep breathing, and reinforces depression. Acupressure can relieve these emotionally based physical symptoms.

Spiritual Practices for Transforming Grief & Sadness

The following acupressure points focus on opening the chest to transform grief and sadness. Sit up comfortably in a chair.

Press Lu 1 (Letting Go): Cross your arms in front of your chest. Use all your fingertips to feel for tension in the upper, outer portion of your chest. Apply firm pressure with your fingers curved. Breathe slowly and deeply for at least one minute. Holding this point can release tears and thus free your spirit.

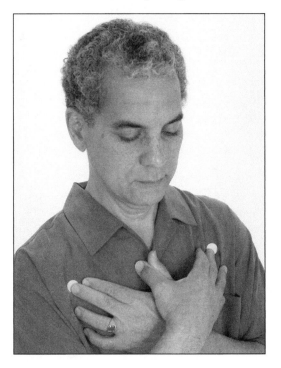

Firmly Touch K 25, K 26, & K 27: Place your fingertips below your throat, at the head of your collarbones. Move your fingers down three rib spaces beside your breastbone.

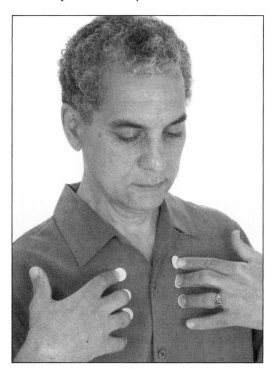

Place your index, middle, and ring fingertips in the indentations between the ribs to stimulate these emotional healing points. Curve your fingers and hold firmly for two minutes as you breathe slowly and deeply. These are very powerful spiritual points for opening the heart and the emotions.

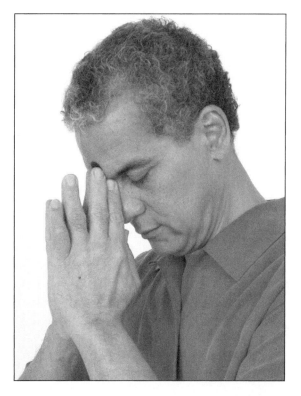

Third Eye Meditation: End by placing your palms together with your middle finger-tips gently touching your Third Eye point (GV 24.5). Meditate on where you are touching as you breathe deeply for two minutes.

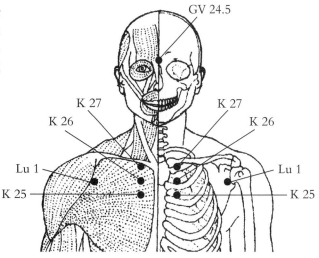

Honoring Yourself

As you grow more sensitive to guidance from the intuitive feelings within, you will gain a sense of knowing what you need to do in any situation. Your intuitive power is always available to guide you whenever you need it.

— Shakti Gawain
Living in the Light

Choose to follow your dreams and aspirations for your highest good. Breathe deeply, go within and explore what is holding you back. Have the courage to face whatever is blocking your heart and spirit. Take a few minutes to explore how you can honor yourself.

Honor yourself by...

- Eating healthy, nutritious foods

- Exercising daily and doing good things for your body

- Practicing meditation, prayer, yoga, or tai chi

- Being in loving, supportive relationships

- Expressing yourself creatively

- Speaking your truth and being assertive about what you need for your spirit to flourish

- Loving and nurturing yourself

- Following your passion and intuition

- Continuing to learn and grow

In your inner journey, don't be afraid of making mistakes; there are no mistakes. Don't be afraid of feeling too much; thank yourself for being capable of experiencing such depth. Be patient with your emotional healing process, which usually involves taking three steps forward and two steps back. Don't let these two steps back into your old negative patterns discourage you; instead, learn from them.

Set your intention to heal from past wounds. Keep your intention alive by nurturing your heart and cultivating your personal growth. Each healing experience will enable you to unravel your emotional pain and will help set you free from the past forever.

You can heal your emotions further by exploring early childhood memories and feelings related to trauma and abuse. The following inner child work is invaluable for deepening acupressure's emotional balancing process.

HEALING THE INNER CHILD

Not having that little girl in your life means you have lost something. You have not had access to her softness, to her sense of trust and wonder. When you hate the child within, you're hating a part of yourself. It is only in taking care of her that you can really learn to take care of yourself. And although you may start with feelings of mistrust and ambivalence, part of healing is accepting her as a part of you.

— Ellen Bass & Laura Davis
The Courage to Heal

Profound emotional and sexual healing can occur if you cultivate a relationship with the part of yourself that was once a child. This child within you, your inner child, knows your emotional needs. Communicating with your inner child about traumatic events can be surprisingly therapeutic.

What happened to you in the past is still a part of you; you're the same person. Let yourself visualize what you looked like or felt as a little girl or boy. What was real then is real now; the memory is inside you. If you choose not to deal with it, the emotional pain from your childhood will remain unconscious. If you find that terror and emotional pain are involved, choose a psychotherapist to provide emotional support to bring your pain into the light by exploring your past. You don't deserve to carry the burden of these awful past experiences. Breathe deeply into your belly to gain the courage to face the unknown; there are many layers to uncover.

Dealing with emotional pain is much more rewarding than holding it in your body. Carrying emotional baggage drains your vitality and prevents you from being able to love fully. Deep emotional scars keep your spirit from soaring, hampering your creativity, alive-ness, and self-esteem. You are in control of how far you go on this journey…

Inner Child Healing Journey

An excellent way to be guided on the following journey is to read the instructions aloud into a tape recorder. As you play it back, you can go more deeply into healing your inner self.

Stage 1:
Creating a Relationship with Your Inner Child

Begin by making yourself comfortable (sitting or lying down) with your eyes closed. Take several slow, deep breaths, through your nose if possible. Place your fingers on your temples in the hollows just outside your eyebrows. Visualize yourself during the time of your childhood trauma or abuse… Notice details about yourself: your hair… your face… your clothing… Also recall the environment you grew up in: your bedroom… your parents' room… the pictures on the wall… the kitchen… your backyard… Breathe deeply into your body for a couple of minutes… Explore whatever feelings or images come to you…

Imagine a photograph taken of you when you were a child… Once you are able to hold an image of what you looked like, say hello to the little girl or boy… Breathe deeply as you notice how your inner child responds… Tell him or her, "I love you"… Breathe deeply as you notice the child's response…

Be aware of the resistance or doubts that surface… Love yourself for what you're going through, whether you see this image of yourself vividly or vaguely, whether he or she is responding to you or not. Acknowledge you were once this child and that he or she is still a part of you…

Breathe deeply into any feelings that are coming up now… Whenever you are afraid, endangered, angry, or traumatized, your inner child will play an important role to guide you… He or she has experienced these feelings far more directly and strongly as a child, and thus carries a wisdom and guidance that can greatly help you heal your emotional wounds…

Breathe deeply, sending loving thoughts as you visualize yourself as a child. Show you care by touching the child within affectionately… Visualize yourself coming closer, on the same level as the child… Notice his or her facial expressions… what the child is doing or communicating…

Take several deep breaths… Realize how you were once this child… Now gradually embrace him or her as you breathe into your heart… Let yourself become this child… Breathe deeply, knowing the attention you give the child is actually a powerful way of loving yourself… Acknowledge your connection with your inner child; your care and attention can cultivate a renewed trust.

Stage 2:
Preparing for the Inner Child Journey

Create a sacred space, a warm, secure environment that feels especially safe. Take the time to prepare the room. You may want a special blanket, pillows, candles, your old flannel pajamas, robe, teddy bear—whatever can support closeness with your inner child.

Begin by making yourself comfortable, holding both Lu 1 points, crossing your forearms over your chest with the heel of one hand on the center of your breastbone to press CV 17. Breathe deeply into your heart for a minute to gather your courage, and let yourself relax as you visualize the child within you…

Now kneel or sit down on a pillow, level with your inner child so he or she will be responsive and comfortable with you… Continue to breathe deeply… Since your inner child knows details and can recall images that may have been difficult for you to remember, ask the child to take you to revisit a very important place. Explain to your inner child that although revisiting this place may be difficult, the journey is necessary to release and heal the past. Assure the child that you are ready and will take special care of him or her and hold hands the whole time.

Ask your inner child if he or she is ready to go on the journey… Breathe deeply as you watch and listen to your inner child… If he or she is ready to go and you are too, move into Stage 3 of this healing journey. If not, ask, "What do you need? When will you be ready?" Continue playing until your inner child is ready to go on the journey…

Stage 3:
Inner Child Journey★

Once you establish a comfortable relationship with your inner child, you are ready for the next step... Have several symbols, tools, or games to play with... Lie down and make yourself comfortable, placing one hand over your belly (CV 6) and the fingers of your other hand on the center of your breastbone to press CV 17. Let your body completely relax as you visualize your inner child...

Breathe deeply into your belly... Continue to gently press the acupressure points on your chest and belly as you imagine holding your inner child's hand. Explore your childhood memories of long ago... Remember to breathe deeply into your heart where you are holding your breastbone.

Visualize a memorable picture of yourself as a child. Ask the child within you to show you where you were hurt... Acknowledge the child for how much he or she remembers... Breathe slowly and deeply into your body as you ask your inner child how the abuse occurred. Explore your feelings and the memories that surface as you ask yourself what your hurt was all about...

Breathe deeply into your lower back to face your fear and pain... Release any pain by opening your mouth and letting the pain out by making a sound. If you feel safe, magnify any feelings or images about a childhood trauma to fully reexperience and release the pain. Breathe love into your heart, loving yourself for what you're going through... You do not need to carry this pain; let it come out of your body...

Breathe deeply into your chest and abdomen... Be aware of any body sensations such as constriction in your throat... Focus on breathing into any tightness or pain... Again, make a sound, exhaling any pain out of you.

Take another deep breath and turn toward your inner child... Acknowledge him or her... Notice what the child's face is saying to you as you look into his or her eyes... Take a mental snapshot ... Use this picture symbolically to empower yourself. You can get a reading on the best ways to give yourself emotional support by visualizing how your inner child responds.

Now embrace the child and stroke his or her head lovingly. Breathe deeply into your belly and tell the child within, "I will never forget you; I will always love you. You are a blessing of the universe; your love and healing came to me to set you free. You are a blessing to me!"

Immediately after the Inner Child Healing Journey, cover yourself with a blanket and take a nap for at least half an hour. This deep relaxation will allow the energy in your body to flow through the meridians to integrate this powerful healing experience. After the deep relaxation, be sure to write down what you experienced in your journal. Writing down the insights, images, and realizations from your journey will substantiate long-lasting emotional healing.

We believe the art of self-acupressure can support your healing and significantly heighten humanity. Time and practice are necessary for allowing healing energy to transform the inner world of your emotions...

★*Caution:* If your emotions are unstable or you have uncontrollable anxieties, go on this part of the journey only with the support of a qualified psychotherapist.

Miracles occur when you live your life with an open heart.

Trust your perceptions and feelings.

As you let go of old confining patterns, your options open.

Remember that perseverance brings great rewards.

Have faith and patience.

Keep your focus on your aspirations

And open your heart to what is right.

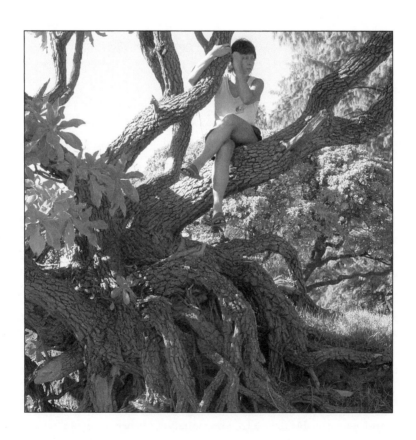

3

GUIDELINES FOR EMOTIONAL BALANCING

We can begin to heal our lives at the deepest levels when we begin to value our bodies and honor their messages instead of feeling victimized by them… Covering up our symptoms with external 'cures' prevents us from 'healing' the parts of our lives that need attention and change.

— Christiane Northrup, MD
Women's Bodies, Women's Wisdom

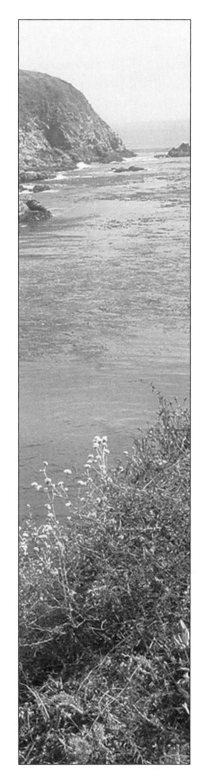

Among the many advantages of acupressure is its safety—even if you have never done it before. Simply follow the instructions, and pay attention to the specific cautions provided. Acupressure is also an excellent treatment for spouses and partners to offer each other and for parents to give to their children for minor problems. Many people choose to work with a certified acupressurist, shiatsu practitioner, or massage therapist, all of whom use the principles of acupressure points and meridians presented in this book. Since acupressure can help heal specific ailments, many massage therapists use acupressure points in their work. So within these pages, psychotherapists, counselors, and health care professionals can find information about how to guide clients using points and deep breathing, and how to end an acupressure routine with deep relaxation to fully integrate the experience.

We highly recommend that you work with a psychotherapist to complement the self-care techniques in this book. Since acupressure is so powerful for releasing emotions, a psychotherapist can support the depth of your emotional healing as you practice the self-care techniques for common emotional complaints in

Part II and for physical complaints in Part III.

Trust is essential for your emotional well-being and for listening to the wisdom of your body. Emotional awareness and discernment empower you to act wisely. Trusting yourself is difficult when you do not have trusting relationships and emotional support. But by developing a keen awareness of your body, breathing into your feelings, and using self-acupressure, you can cultivate the courage you need to embrace your healing journey.

The Buddha gained enlightenment by observing and watching his thoughts and feelings without allowing himself to be overcome by them. Balance comes from being in the present moment and trusting yourself to act on your feelings. Once you identify your feelings, you can use your better judgment to sort out what feels right and act accordingly.

Acupressure's healing touch can increase your awareness of your feelings and of the area being touched. When the points are held, emotions stored in the body often come to the surface. When a sore point is held, a surge of emotion such as joy or fear may release laughter or tears. Pressing points can enable you to become more aware of the tensions being held in your body and facilitate the release of your emotions.

Emotions are like water. Some people release them spontaneously, like the gush and spray of a waterfall; others need more time and a strong sense of trust, and no distractions before their emotional wave can crest. Accept your feelings and what they are expressing. For instance, fear expresses your limitations and boundaries of the unknown. Fear is healthy when it signals caution or danger; it is out of balance and unhealthy when it provokes excessive paranoia or denial.

How often have you heard someone say to a small child, "Don't cry" or "Don't feel sad"? While the parent may believe she is protecting her child from hurt, in truth these statements lead to shutting down feelings. These are terrible messages to teach a child at any age. Imagine, if we taught our children instead to become aware of their feelings through reflection and meditation; they would also learn how to be aware of thoughts and actions connected to those feelings.

Body Messages

To know the truth of the body is to be aware of its movements, its impulses and its restraints, that is, to feel what goes on in the body. If an individual doesn't feel the tensions, rigidities, or anxieties, (s)he is, in this sense, denying the truth of the body.

— Alexander Lowen
Love and Orgasm

Your emotions and your body awareness are a direct communication system. Your body communicates what you need through your emotions, sending signals for your body's well-being. Different emotions or thoughts create specific responses and symptoms. For instance, suppose you feel irritated by someone's obtrusive comments or lack of boundaries. When you listen to your body and speak your truth, your courage to be assertive may transform the intruder into someone who can respond to your expressed needs.

The lower back, home to the kidneys and adrenal glands, is affected by fear and phobias. Rising fear activates the adrenal glands.

Emotional body responses can also be unpredictable and complex. Shoulder tension, for example, can be caused by anger, fear, stress, or anxiety, among other things. Anxiety or sadness may cause your chest to contract, worry may cause your jaw muscles to ache, and anger may cause your stomach to knot up. Unresolved emotional experiences become rooted subconsciously in your body.

Within the body there are places where memories are stored that we are often unaware of but that, through acupressure, we can bring into consciousness. Every unexpressed emotion creates its own internal chemical and physical response. The longer feelings remain unexpressed, the greater the likelihood they will cause physical problems within the body. Thus, the body's messages reflect the internal dialogue of the emotions.

Types of Awareness

Your body is a tremendous helper in learning to follow your inner voice. Whenever it is in pain or discomfort, it is usually an indication that you have ignored your feelings. Use it as a signal to tune in and ask what you need to be aware of.

— Shakti Gawain
Living in the Light

There are three types of awareness: outer awareness, inner awareness, and fantasy. Outer awareness is awareness of what you see, smell, hear, and feel through external touch. Awareness of images, sounds, and smells can trigger memories and feelings. Inner awareness is awareness of sensations underneath the surface of the skin, such as your heartbeat, abdominal discomfort, or a lump in your throat. It includes noticing grief, sadness, anger, anxiety, fear, or joyful feelings. Fantasy involves imagination and intuition.

Your outer awareness can distract you from focusing on your inner awareness. For instance, touch can distract you from or enhance inner awareness, depending on how it is applied. The sensory experience of being touched can divert your attention from your emotions; when you're about to cry and someone rubs or pats your back, the physical contact may distract you, making it difficult to go within and release your tears. But being held in an embrace or holding an acupressure point is contact that supports an emotional release. Such conscious touch can enhance your inner awareness.

When you practice the self-care routines in this book, say to yourself, "Now, I am aware of…" and finish the sentence. Notice which of the three types of awareness come to you, and see if there is a pattern. Many insights can come from working with this simple exercise while practicing self-acupressure.

Modes of Perception

Guiding awareness involves working with four modes of perception: seeing, hearing, thinking, and feeling. Each mode uses a different sense of experience. One of these modes often dominates how a person learns and accesses information.

Utilizing your primary mode can cultivate emotional healing. If sight is your predominant mode, using visualizations in your healing work will be the most beneficial. If you are sensitive to sound, transformation can occur through listening to affirmations or your inner voice. If you have a strong intellect, journaling may help you process your thoughts to release whatever is causing your emotional distress. If you learn best from doing, working actively with your body awareness can be most beneficial for your emotional growth.

Sometimes you will need to let go of what appears to be your strength for a less familiar mode. If you are intellectual, exploring your body sensations can bring about new insights. If you are right-handed, drawing with your left hand can bring out your vulnerabilities and unexpressed feelings. By shifting into a foreign mode, you can experience another depth of perception for transforming your problems.

SELF-CARE GUIDELINES

As you enter your body more fully, you become aware of a new sense of emotional being, a new connectedness with life. You become one with your body, and simultaneously one with your experience. Emotional growth coincides with your connection to your body.

— John Ruskan
Emotional Clearing

Focus on Deep Breathing: Deep breathing nourishes an emotional release as water nurtures a garden. The increased oxygen heightens your senses as well as your capacity to feel. Thus, be sure to consciously remind yourself to breathe deeply. The more slowly and deeply you breathe, the calmer you will feel. Inspire yourself to take full, complete breaths to facilitate your healing process. Maintain awareness of your breath at all times while practicing acupressure.

Practice Body Awareness & Go Within: Create a private area free of distractions, and set aside the time needed, to go deep within. Your inner experience will become amplified, and you will have greater insight, when your eyes are closed. Feel your body; breathe deeply, and notice what images or feelings arise.

Be Present & Aware of Your Physical Body: When past memories or distressful feelings surface, return to the present moment by breathing slowly and deeply. As you do so, feel your body to ground your experience. Wiggle your toes… shake your shoulders gently… squeeze your buttocks and take slow deep breaths into your body.

Focus on Your Body to Get at the Source of the Problem: While you breathe deeply into your body, visualize the source of your emotional pain, and ask yourself, "What is this pain telling me?" Allow yourself time to explore your body's signals and its wisdom. Healing a traumatic experience involves both insight and the reexperience of your feelings.

Apply Acupressure Therapy: As you hold the points, breathing deeply can enhance your emotional sensitivity. Holding points without any movement is most effective for fostering an emotional release. The stillness allows you to deeply relax and explore feelings without being distracted by massage strokes. Touch increases body awareness. When your eyes are closed, your awareness becomes focused on where you are touched. For example, by placing your hand on your lower belly, you can become more aware of intestinal congestion and whatever feelings are stored in this area. Deep relaxation from receiving acupressure can also release memories, feelings, and a wide variety of involuntary body responses such as shaking, yawning, or a light, spacey feeling. As points are held, the flow of healing energy increases, memories become more vivid, and feelings easily surface. Whenever you need to calm or settle your feelings in the emotional healing process, use all of your fingertips to press the Sea of Tranquility (CV 17), in the indentations on the center of your breastbone.

Be Aware of Your Limitations: If you are feeling ungrounded or unstable, you may need the outside support of a counselor or therapist, especially when you experience the following:

- **Uncontrollable emotions,** fantasies, or memories

- **Recurring anxiety,** fear, depression, nightmares, or rage

- **Suicidal thoughts** and tendencies

- **Confusion** and instability

Visualize Your Connection with the Earth: Imagine a grounding cord connecting the base of your spine with the center of the earth. For protection, visualize your body being surrounded by white or golden light.

Cover Yourself: After an emotional release, your body may shake, release tears, or feel chilled. Be sure to cover yourself or wear warm clothing after receiving acupressure, and pay special attention to your body needs.

Guiding Others in Self-Acupressure

If you are guiding someone else on holding their acupressure points, continue to give them deep breathing instructions and stay focused in the present moment. The first step to increasing inner awareness is deep relaxation. Create a safe environment and establish trust in a comfortable position. Instruct your partner to use self-massage for a few minutes on any tight muscles and encourage long, slow deep breathing.

Continue to guide your partner to breathe deeply as she holds two acupressure points steady, without moving. When a point releases and the tension surrounding the point softens or begins to pulse regularly, move to another point. Apply pressure gradually and firmly. Your finger pressure should not be so deep as to elicit an uncomfortable pain or soreness. Instead, the intention of your touch is to increase your body awareness. Maintain a presence in your fingertips similar to the experience of being held and completely supported.

Guide your partner to relax and breathe deeply into the chest or belly. Most emotional wounds, memories, and responses get stored in this part of the body. The throat, buttocks, and genitals are other common areas where emotions are stored. While holding acupressure points, guide your partner to pay attention to all body sensations and feelings, no matter how subtle or vague.

The words you use to guide the self-care will depend on what mode of awareness your partner favors. Find out your partner's main mode by asking, "Do you learn best from listening, seeing, feeling, or doing? Is your strongest experience visual, intellectual, auditory, or body oriented?" If your partner is visual, she may tell you what she is seeing. If she is kinesthetic—that is, highly attuned to the movements of her body—she may tell you about a sensory feeling. If she is more mentally oriented, she may share her thoughts. If she is more auditory, she might be more inclined to tell you about the various sounds she notices. Listen for the language she uses, to increase the value of the session.

Once your partner expresses what she is experiencing (even if she reports that nothing is going on), acknowledge what you heard by feeding back her words to redescribe the experience. If she feels tired, encourage her to breathe deeply into the fatigue. If she feels angry, encourage her to breathe consciously and deeply into the anger. Again, acknowledge what you have heard by using her words to describe the experience. This form of active listening enables her to further focus on her inner experience. Do not go off on a tangent; do not express what you think her images or feelings mean. This would be a distraction. Instead, stay with her inner experience.

Give your partner enough time and encouragement to explore whatever is coming up for her. Acknowledge her feelings. If she reports

stomach pain, you might say, "Breathe deeply into that pain and explore what it's connected to...." This will encourage deep breathing to uncover the source of the pain. After guiding her through a self-acupressure session, be sure to use the guidelines below to deeply relax and assimilate the healing energy.

After Receiving Acupressure

Close your eyes…
Begin long deep breathing and
Let yourself completely relax from head to toe…

As you breathe,
Tell each part of your body to relax…

Be good to yourself; enjoy letting yourself go…
As your thoughts and feelings surface…
Love yourself for what you are going through.

How you treat yourself after receiving acupressure will affect your energy flow and your emotional well-being. Deep relaxation is essential immediately after receiving a full session. The longer and deeper the points are pressed, the longer you should relax. If you work on a full self-care routine for ten to fifteen minutes, a few additional minutes of deep relaxation with your eyes closed is optimal. But if you spend more time stimulating points and have an emotional experience, be sure to:

- Deeply relax immediately afterward, cover yourself, and take a nap to maximize the flow of healing energy through the points.

- Avoid cold drinks and icy foods.

- Try to avoid hectic environments or tense situations for twenty-four hours. Your system is more vulnerable and can absorb whatever stress is in your surroundings.

If you cannot relax immediately after a session, be sure to plan time later to deeply relax. Once you get to a secure, comfortable place to unwind, spend a few minutes stretching to relax your muscles. After stretching, immediately lie down on your back with your spine supported and your head in alignment. Cover yourself with a blanket and get cozy, take slow breaths, and relax deeply.

How to Integrate an Emotional Healing Session

After taking a nap or giving yourself at least ten minutes to completely relax, practice the following activities to integrate your emotional healing session and come back to daily life refreshed:

- **Rotate your wrists and ankles** for one minute as you breathe deeply.

- **Massage your feet** thoroughly including your ankles, heels, arches, foot bottoms, and the toes for a couple minutes.

- **Briskly rub St 36** on both sides. Make fists, and place them on the outside of both legs just below your knees. Use your fists to briskly rub up and down along the outside of your shinbones. Encourage yourself to breathe deeply as you stimulate these points for one minute.

These instructions are effective for grounding yourself and rejuvenating the body's energy system after an emotional healing session. If you still feel tired, weak, or unstable, be sure to go back into a longer and deeper relaxation period—preferably give yourself a nurturing nap to renew your mind, body, and spirit.

In addition to deep relaxation, many other techniques can further complement acupressure. The next chapter provides guidelines for working with a psychotherapist and other activities that can further cultivate emotional balancing.

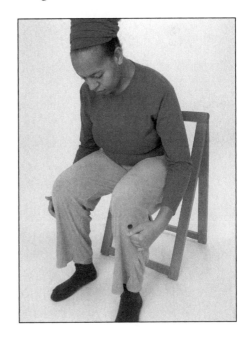

4

EMOTIONAL SUPPORT

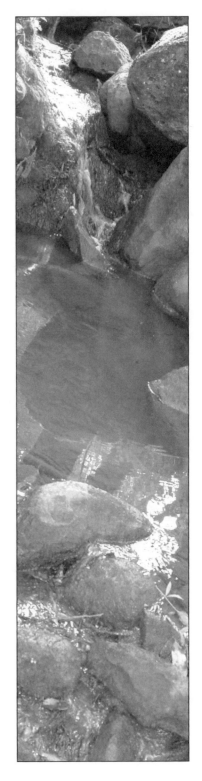

The more you can accept your feelings without judgment, the easier it will be for you to experience them, work with them, and learn from them.

— Ellen Bass & Laura Davis
The Courage to Heal

This chapter offers resources and suggestions for personal growth activities and therapies that enhance the self-care acupressure routines in this book. First, you will learn the importance of using deep breathing during an emotional release. Second, we will help you choose the right psychotherapist to further assist your self-healing. We highly recommend that you work with a psychotherapist as a complement to support the depth of your emotional healing as you practice the self-care techniques for common complaints. Third, psychotherapists and bodyworkers will receive special guidance for integrating acupressure and supporting their clients.

Deep Breathing:
Support for Emotional Release

Emotional healing involves exploring the unknown. Facing unfamiliar territory can cause fears to arise. How you respond to these fears can be pivotal for your personal growth. Overwhelming feelings can be scary and paralyze your ability to respond. These same awesome feelings can also be exhilarating and inspiring when you trust yourself and have faith that your body won't betray you. Self-acupressure provides a safe, reassuring connection with your body when you are facing stressful experiences and relaxes you so that you do not become petrified with intense emotions and memories.

Shallow breathing often occurs when fears arise, contracting your body and obstructing your senses. When you breathe shallowly, the cells of your body do not get enough oxygen to be fully nourished. As a result, your inner awareness, sensory perceptions, and intuition decrease.

Your breath flow is crucial for obtaining the full benefits of the emotional healing process. Oxygen is essential for exploring uncharted emotional territory. The more deeply you breathe, the more deeply you can go in your healing journey.

We encourage you to learn how to breathe slowly and deeply while you practice the self-care routines in this book, so you can handle the powerful feelings that may arise. Whenever an intense emotional upheaval occurs, be sure to breathe slowly and deeply through your nose. Rapid and deep breathing through your mouth can lead to hyperventilation. To prevent hyperventilation, simply close your mouth and breathe slowly.

Your breath can be used as a safety valve when you feel off-kilter or in distress. Acupressure on CV 17, in the indentation on the center of your breastbone, can regulate your breathing; it has a calming effect and relieves hyperventilation almost instantly. Holding CV 17 while you do slow, deep breathing in and out of your nose will regulate the amount of air you assimilate; it is an excellent technique for calming anxiety and nervousness.

Your body registers multiple reactions during a traumatic experience. The experience of a car accident may last for only a few seconds, but your senses will absorb the sounds, visual images, thoughts, feelings, and the tremendous impact on your body. Your body stores trauma in muscle tissue, commonly in your back muscles.

The back, however, is difficult to reach on yourself; you will want a partner to hold your back points or else lie on tennis balls for several minutes. While your back tension releases, buried trauma, emotional pain, and other memories often arise.

Reliving the experience and releasing associated emotional pain during a session can free the trauma from your body. Releasing traumatic burdens often creates profound spiritual experiences such as radiant light or streams of warmth flowing through your body.

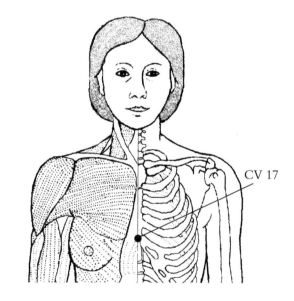

CV 17

Acupressure & Psychotherapy

The quality of health care depends not only on how well physicians and other health professionals perform their tasks and the reliability of the technologies they use but also on their ability to be human. To touch and be touched is part of the process of staying well or getting well.

— John G. Bruhn, PhD
Southern Medical Journal

Acupressure complements psychotherapy by working somatically with both the mind and body. When a psychotherapy client is tense, body awareness, intuition, recollection, and the ability to visualize are blocked. Increased benefits result from working with both acupressure and psychotherapy. Having a bodyworker relax a client in preparation for psychotherapy can profoundly enhance the healing session. At the end of therapy, an acupressurist can balance the client by holding specific points to integrate whatever was dealt with in the session.

While in psychotherapy, clients may process many unresolved issues, past relationships, and traumatic experiences. Some people discover that thinking about their issues causes them to get "stuck inside their head." Excessive mental processing can be counterproductive and lead to headaches and other physical complaints. When the dynamics of the mind and body are imbalanced (which often occurs in the best bodywork or talk therapies), the client becomes disoriented or continues their self-abusive patterns. Acupressure in conjunction

with psychotherapy can help the client integrate the personal insights attained in therapy. This book offers a series of acupressure points specifically recommended for grounding a client in therapy (see page 43).

Choosing the Right Psychotherapist

Counseling is not always comfortable, but you know you're with a good counselor when you develop more and more skills to heal yourself as time goes on. You become able to recognize your own patterns and to feel and interpret your own emotions.

— Ellen Bass & Laura Davis
The Courage to Heal

Talk therapy or counseling sessions for processing life's challenges can be a great asset for personal growth. Psychotherapy with a skilled therapist can foster emotional healing. A compassionate, sensitive psychotherapist or counselor can give you support to deal with issues and provide guidance for practicing the exercises in this book. Look for a psychotherapist who:

• Facilitates self-discovery and supports self-awareness during the healing process

• Helps you integrate behavior, emotions, and feelings with body awareness

• Models healthy boundaries and behaviors in client relationships

• Is attentive to your body's wisdom using both verbal and nonverbal messages

- Supports your inner journey to safely explore childhood traumatic memories

- Provides a safe environment to let out loud sounds for expressing any grief or anger

- Uses body language and facial expressions to give you feedback and encouragement

The first step in counseling is to establish the trust needed to explore personal feelings and issues. Trust cultivates a person's willingness to express and share their vulnerabilities. Emotional healing cannot fully take place unless a person has the trust and willpower to make positive life changes.

Select a therapist whose philosophy seems most likely to facilitate your personal growth. Some therapists use guided imagery and hypnosis or voice dialogue; others use role-playing, dreamwork, psychosynthesis, breathwork, art therapy, authentic moment, cathartic therapy, and talk therapy. Many humanistic and transpersonal psychotherapists, who may be members of the Association of Humanistic Psychology (AHP) or the Association of Transpersonal Psychology (ATP), use a creative mix of several of these modalities, including active listening, depending upon their clients' needs. A growing number of therapists practice somatic psychotherapy or utilize mind/body/spirit approaches. You may not know what suits you best until you try some of these different approaches.

Choose a therapist you feel comfortable working with. Some therapists will simply listen, support, and empathize; some may offer suggestions and give advice; while others may challenge you. The best way to find a therapist you feel good working with is to shop around and compare different therapy styles and individual personalities.

Suggestions for Psychotherapists

This book can complement psychotherapy in many ways. You can give clients self-care routines for working on themselves at home. As issues, memories, or images surface through self-acupressure, clients can work on those experiences in their next psychotherapy session.

You can also guide clients to hold specific acupressure points, which will enable them to access their unresolved issues more easily. Self-acupressure heightens body awareness by opening the circulation of blood and energy through the points. Awareness is key to transforming psychological blocks and altering behavior. Many psychotherapists are surprised to discover how easily and effectively they are able to integrate their counseling and therapeutic skills with acupressure. Many therapists themselves have found this somatic approach to be profoundly transformational.

This book contains an integration of various somatic techniques for your clients. Using self-acupressure as an adjunct to therapy along with breathwork, visualization, and healing affirmations can heighten your therapeutic process. When you have a client who is stuck and unable to move through their problems, you may find the acupressure techniques in this book effective to facilitate a transformational breakthrough.

Suggestions for Bodyworkers

Emotional releases often occur spontaneously during bodywork. Bodyworkers with knowledge of the proper acupressure points can be of enormous service to their clients. Knowing the scope and limits of your practice is vitally important. Cultivate referral relationships with psychotherapists who you believe are well equipped to handle difficult or frightening feelings and issues that could arise during bodywork.

This book can provide massage therapists with coping tools, acupressure points, and self-care routines for clients to work on emotional issues at home. Providing these resources adds value to your massage sessions. Learning acu-pressure is a natural next step for many massage therapists. Acupressure will tremendously benefit your hands-on practice in rewarding ways. You will be able to relieve common ailments such as headaches, backache, pain, insomnia, nausea, and carpal tunnel as well as balance the emotions. (See Appendix D in the back of this book for information on acupressure training programs.)

EMOTIONAL BALANCING POINTS FOR THERAPISTS

The following acupressure points are useful for bodyworkers and psychotherapists to incorporate into their private practice:

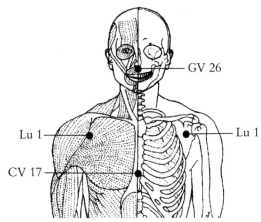

- **Center of the Person** (GV 26, located between the upper lip and nose): Apply pressure firmly into the upper gum. Use this famous first-aid revival point when you find your client's eyes fluttering and rolling back or notice other indications that the client may be losing consciousness. Holding this point is also good for relieving dizziness and stabilizing an emotional release.

- **Sea of Tranquility** (CV 17, located on the center of the breastbone): This is the best point to hold during an emotional release for calming your client. Also use this point for relieving anxiety, panic attacks, and nervousness. Hold the Sea of Tranquility to calm yourself and make deep breathing easier.

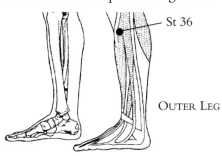

OUTER LEG

- **Letting Go** (Lu 1, located on the upper, outer part of the chest): This point is excellent for grieving and processing feelings. Holding it facilitates emotional release and is also good for releasing depression and expectations.

- **Three Mile** (St 36, located four finger-widths below the knee, outside the shinbone): St 36 is the most effective point to enable a client to come back into their body after an emotional release. This point is also energizing.

COMPLEMENTARY THERAPIES & ACTIVITIES

Daily Exercise

We recommend aerobic exercise, weight-bearing routines, and stretching such as yoga or Pilates. Aerobic exercise—such as jogging, brisk walking, swimming, and bicycling—effectively improves the body's physical and emotional stamina. Weight-bearing exercises build strength. Feeling stronger is especially empowering for victims of abuse. Stretching increases circulation and flexibility.

The word *aerobic* pertains to the free circulation of air for stimulating respiration. Performing strenuous exercise for fifteen to twenty minutes strengthens and fully oxygenates the cardiovascular system. When the cells of your body receive more oxygen, you naturally feel better. Studies on exercise programs show an increase in vitality, self-confidence, and improvement in participants' self-image.★

Vigorous aerobic exercise, such as power walking, running, cycling, or swimming, for at least thirty minutes increases endorphin levels. Endorphins are natural body chemicals that mediate pain and create euphoria when the body is highly stimulated. Based on recent research studies at top universities, experts say that the strong effect that exercise has on mood makes it an essential component in relieving mild to moderate depression. People who exercise daily and take care of their bodies seem to have a better overall feeling about themselves and their lives.

Positive Thinking

Thinking positively may have a strong effect on how you feel about yourself and others. Many researchers have studied the long-term effects of negative thinking and pessimism on minor and major health conditions. Some studies have shown that a judgmental or self-critical attitude can contribute to headaches, hypertension, and other ailments.

Worry and preoccupation with your daily problems can cause you to miss wonderful opportunities before you. Appreciating what you have helps develop an attitude of gratitude.

Keep a gratitude journal to cultivate awareness of what is going right in your life. Record three things that you are grateful for each day. In this way, natural miracles can become common, everyday occurrences.

Meditation & Prayer

The ancient practices of prayer and meditation are especially complementary to acupressure. When you pray or meditate while holding the points, you can further develop your connection with the healing energy of your body and the universe. By studying meditation practices, researchers are discovering that mindfulness meditation can bring about positive changes in brain activity and the immune system.

Prayer and meditation are powerful ways to ask for guidance. Prayer connects your dreams and aspirations with all of creation. Instead of being limited in your thinking, prayer and faith offer infinite possibilities.

★Kenneth Cooper, MD, MPH, *The Aerobics Program for Total Well-Being, The Complete Guide to Your Emotions and Your Health* (Emmaus, PA: Rodale Press, 1992), 21–25.

Often people go through the day unaware of their thoughts and actions. Stress and anxiety cloud their thoughts and are obstacles to cultivating the inner awareness essential for achieving emotional balance. The calming effects of meditation can clear your thoughts and also cultivate the inner awareness essential for emotional balance. To change a negative emotion, first become aware of your feelings and your intention to change. Then use meditation to clear your mind and gain a new perspective.

Meditation Guidelines

- **Posture:** Sit comfortably with your spine straight. Keep your chin slightly tucked in. Place your hands comfortably in your lap, cupped one over the other. There are many other hand positions or *mudras* you can use to meditate for emotional balancing.

- **Time:** Have a clock nearby to keep track of your meditation time. Start with just five minutes. Choose to meditate for the full five minutes without moving. Progressively build up to ten minutes, then fifteen and finally twenty. Mornings and just before retiring at night are excellent times to meditate. A regular meditation schedule is helpful to solidify your practice.

- **Stillness:** Be as still as possible when you meditate. If you have an itch, try not to scratch and watch the sensation pass. Observe yourself, your feelings, and your breath. If you want to scratch, do so with awareness, not automatically. Training yourself to be conscious creates profound changes in your thoughts, words, and actions. Make intentional choices without being attached to your thoughts.

Breathing Meditation

Hold CV 17 in the center of your breastbone, four finger-widths above the base of the breastbone, as you begin the following deep breathing meditation.

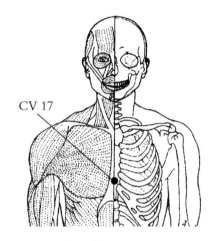

CV 17

Find a comfortable sitting position with your spine straight. Take a few deep breaths, and observe your breathing. Pay attention to the smooth rhythm of your inhalations and exhalations. If extraneous thoughts come into your mind, simply be aware of them, then let them go and return your attention to your breath. If you can stay focused on following your breath for three to five minutes, you are off to a very good start.

Meditation is a practice cultivated over time. Observe your thoughts as if they were clouds passing by. As you breathe, say to yourself, "Breathing in, I am aware of my thoughts; breathing out, I let them go." You can also count your breaths from one to ten and then start over again with one. If you get caught up in your thoughts, simply go back to the breath. Be aware of how one thought leads to a whole series of other thoughts and creates a huge drama in your mind. Often this mental drama is played out through words and actions. When a negative attitude, judgment, or expectation dominates your thoughts, become aware of how the scenario began. By becoming aware of your thoughts, you can change them or let them go. The first step is awareness.

Thich Nhat Hanh, a Vietnamese Buddhist monk who has written a number of beautiful books on meditation, teaches the practice of mindfulness. Through mindfulness you learn how everything you do can become a meditation.

Varieties of Meditation

Having a meditation instructor or a group of people to meditate with can be beneficial when you are first learning. There are many ways to meditate and a variety of styles. The most basic is to simply follow the depth of your breath. The following meditation styles can be beneficial for emotional healing:

- **Vipassana Meditation** allows the flow of thoughts to come and go, fostering mental flexibility.

- **Transcendental Meditation (TM)** allows you to connect to the oneness of creation and leads to peace of mind. Giving your mind and body a rest, this form of meditation releases trauma and calms stressful emotions.

- **Yogic Meditation** focuses on breathing and stretching your body in therapeutic postures. Deep breathing expands your awareness and can enable you to stretch even further. Yoga is profoundly relaxing and particularly beneficial to the nervous system.

When someone makes you angry or upset, instead of reacting negatively, send them a positive thought or use a meditation technique such as conscious deep breathing. This will transform negativity and create the opportunity for a positive outcome. Sometimes your worst enemy can be your greatest teacher. Be grateful for the opportunity to learn from the most difficult challenges to your personal growth.

Meditation and prayer can calm your mind and balance your emotions. When practiced regularly with self-acupressure, they can counteract worry, grief, and self-doubt. Praying for world peace and on behalf of people less fortunate is also a positive way to reduce preoccupation with your own worries and stress.

CREATIVE WAYS TO RELEASE TRAUMA

The following therapeutic exercises can help you manage emotional distress and deal with repressed feelings. You will find that they complement each other; each supports a different aspect of the emotional healing process. Some foster reflection for sorting out past traumatic experiences; others facilitate greater awareness of your feelings and your body's responses in the present moment. The main purpose of these exercises is to nurture self-love, trust, safety, and acceptance. They are excellent supplements to the self-acupressure routines in this book and can greatly enhance your emotional healing. As you explore them, note which ones benefit you the most and practice them regularly.

Hands-On Diary

Keep a personal diary of your self-acupressure practice to record your progress. Acupressure effects can be subtle, and you may experience new awarenesses, feelings, and dreams. Sometimes the benefits take a few weeks to notice. Make note of your body's responses to specific points and techniques. Record the points and techniques that helped you most and the amount of time you spent. This account can be valuable for learning about your body's needs for emotional healing.

Use the Hands-On Diary on page 55 or create your own diary. Writing down your feelings, experiences, and memories can itself be a vehicle to express and release trauma. Writing about a traumatic experience will stimulate you to reflect; it can heighten your awareness and validate your experience. Sorting out your memories can be very healing.

Free Association

Writing down what comes to mind or whatever you are feeling can help you access repressed feelings and experiences. If you have resistance to writing, try talking into a mini–tape recorder. The process of freely expressing yourself can release important information for your emotional healing and growth.

Creating sentences to complete can encourage free association. Some examples are:

• What I don't trust is…

• What I really resent is…

• What scares me the most is…

• What I really need to say is…

Autobiographical Experiences

Write down or tape-record the story of your life. You can start from birth, or choose a stressful or traumatic experience to begin with. Reflecting while recounting the details of your experience will open a dynamic healing process. Completing your autobiography can become the basis for uncovering memories and gaining new awareness.

You can also choose a personal issue or highly charged topic to focus on, such as money, childhood issues, or sex. For example, you can reflect on how affection was expressed in your family.

Laura Davis's *The Courage to Heal Workbook,* Kathleen Adams's *Journal to the Self,* and Nathaniel Branden's *If You Could Hear What I Cannot Say* are all books that can help you explore writing as an emotional healing tool (see Selected Bibliography).

Self-Portrait

Art can be a powerful medium to unveil what is unconscious, and it is accessible to many people. It is especially useful with preschool children. A person who is unable to talk or write may be able to express their feelings through art.

A pencil and paper are all you need to get started, but you can use all kinds of materials, such as magazine clippings, clay, paints and crayons. Mask-making with papier-mâché is an excellent medium for getting in touch with and expressing your shadow self.

Try having a dialogue with the art you made—the characters, figures, and shapes. Breathe deeply as you interact with your artwork, and notice what feelings surface. If you have flashbacks, a history of depression, hostile behavior, or emotional instability, be sure to have a trustworthy support person with you.

Body-Oriented Methods

Many techniques utilize the body to access stored traumatic experiences. You can use any combination of movement, self-massage, deep breathing, and guided awareness to explore at your own pace.

Authentic movement is a form of psychotherapy that explores self-expression through body gestures and motions. This body-oriented therapy focuses on behavioral patterns, using movement to make you more aware of unconscious experiences. As you work on your body and new memories or feelings surface, explore other therapeutic methods such as transpersonal, humanistic, or Hakomi psychotherapy, journaling, dialoguing, or drawing to further express yourself.

We believe that incorporating many of these adjunct therapies can further develop your personal growth and increase your awareness. Deep-rooted issues take time to heal. Be loving and patient with yourself. Respect your personal limitations, being careful not to push yourself too far.

PART II:

APPLICATIONS FOR EMOTIONAL IMBALANCES

*Follow your feelings through your defenses to their sources, and
bring to the light… those aspects of yourself that resist wholeness, that
live in fear. The journey to authentic power requires that you become
conscious of all that you feel… Feel your intentions in your heart.
Feel not what your mind tells you, but what your heart tells you.*

— Gary Zukav
The Seat of the Soul

COMMON
EMOTIONAL COMPLAINTS

QUICK REFERENCE GUIDE

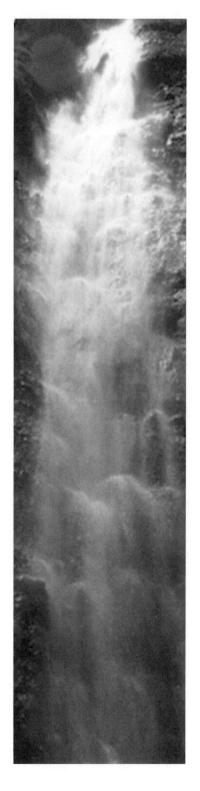

For each chapter topic, you will find:

- **A Brief Introduction to the Emotional Complaint,** its causes, and related issues

- **A Short Story** of how we applied acupressure for a specific complaint

- **Healing Affirmations** for directing your thoughts in a positive way

- **Anatomical Line Drawings,** showing the most effective acupressure points to use

- **Point Descriptions,** with each point's location and benefits

- **Photographs** that illustrate the self-acupressure techniques

- **Quick Tips or a Miniroutine** that is easy to do anywhere

- **Self-Care Routine** with step-by-step instructions of how to best use the points

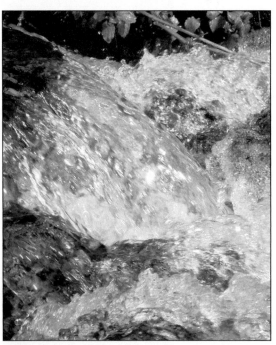

Guidelines for Using Self-Acupressure

The clearer and stronger your intention, the more quickly your creative visualization will work. In any given situation, ask yourself about the condition of your intention.
If it is weak or uncertain, it can often be strengthened by affirming: I now have total intention to create this here and now!

— Shakti Gawain
Creative Visualization

Each acupressure point is effective for relieving multiple complaints. One point, for example, may be good for relieving several emotional imbalances, such as fear, anxiety, depression, and worry. Thus, you will find that many of the points are used repeatedly throughout the book. The point CV 17 (Sea of Tranquility), for instance, is effective for balancing and soothing most emotional upheavals.

For a given ailment or concern, practice the acupressure techniques in the relevant chapter several times to get familiar with them. Once you are accustomed to them, try the shorter miniroutine. It should take only ten minutes, while the longer self-care routine will take approximately thirty minutes. The full self-care routine is most effective when practiced in its entirety, but you can still benefit from using just one or two points. For instance, when you are out in public and get upset, you can easily practice a quick tip or miniroutine to respond immediately. Then when you have more time and privacy, practice the full self-care routine, which covers more points and enables you to go into greater depth for your emotional healing. After you have practiced a self-care routine for over ten minutes, be sure to treat yourself to several minutes of deep relaxation, to obtain the optimal benefits.

The ideal situation for practicing self-acupressure is a quiet, relaxing environment that supports your emotional healing process. Start a self-care routine by gently stretching your body. Reach your arms upward and stretch, as you might do when getting up in the morning. Then gently stretch the back of your legs. Sit comfortably in a chair, or simply lie down on a carpeted floor or on top of your bed to practice the routines.

Most of the self-care routines can also be practiced while at work, sitting in a chair. Sit back with your spine supported, feet flat on the floor, and take several long, deep breaths as you hold the points. With a little creativity or concentration, you can transform any space— even an airport terminal, an office, or an airplane—into a setting suitable for self-acupressure. Headphones can provide you with a symphony of healing sounds. You can also imagine yourself in a relaxed environment at home, in a park, or on a quiet beach, listening to the healing sounds of the waves.

Stimulate the points several times throughout the day for best results, especially for a chronic or intense problem. We recommend you do self-acupressure at least two or three times per day. Even if you practice occasionally, however, you will still derive benefits. Create a consistent practice that works with your schedule and lifestyle. Certainly, the more you practice acupressure, the greater the results.

Breathing Guidelines

As you practice the self-care routines, concentrate on breathing deeply into your abdomen. This will help your body heal itself and generate well-being. Deep breathing enables tension to release, encourages healing energy to flow throughout the body, and can relieve pain. When your breath is shallow, your body's vital systems function at a minimum level. With long, deep breathing the respiratory system functions properly and your cells become fully oxygenated. Deep breathing is especially effective with acupressure for releasing emotional pain.

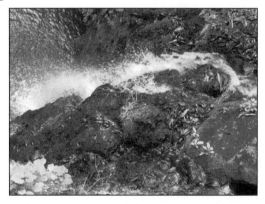

Close your eyes and focus your attention on a painful emotional issue or experience for several minutes... Breathe deeply... Imagine breathing healing energy into your body... Inhale deeply into the abdomen, letting your belly expand... Feel the breath reach into the depths of your belly... Exhale slowly, letting the energy circulate throughout your body...

This basic deep breathing technique will enhance the benefits of all the acupressure routines in this book. Holding acupressure points while taking slow deep breaths closes the pain gates of the nervous system, oxygenates your body, and purifies your blood.

Deep Relaxation Guide

After you practice an acupressure routine from one of the following chapters, follow it immediately with this Deep Relaxation exercise. Be sure to leave yourself at least five to ten minutes for it, to gain its healing benefits.

In the exercise you will focus on each part of your body in turn, utilizing your awareness to cultivate deep relaxation. It is an excellent tool for getting in touch with your body sensations and letting go of emotional pain and tension. Breathe deeply throughout the whole exercise, and consciously tell your body to relax.

To begin, lie down on your back or sit comfortably in a chair. We suggest that you record the instructions, pausing after each sentence, so that you can play it at the end of your acupressure routines.

Close your eyes, and begin by breathing into your heart… Feel your body relax… Wiggle your toes and let them relax… Rotate your feet and tell your ankles to relax… Gently move your legs, feeling your calves, knees, and thighs relax… Tighten your buttock muscles, and then let them relax… Feel your abdominal organs and pelvic area relax… Take several long, slow, deep breaths into your abdominal area, letting your belly relax… Whatever you are holding on to inside your mind, just let it go…

Now feel your whole back and let it relax… Relax your arms… and each finger… Tell your shoulders and neck to relax… Let go of any tension in your forehead… Let your temples and ears relax… Move your jaw from side to side, letting it relax… Relax your nose and your throat… Bring your attention to your eyes, and let them rest… Feel your whole body relax… Allow your thoughts to flow… Let yourself completely relax…

During deep relaxation your whole consciousness changes. When you are completely relaxed, your mind is able to experience oneness with your body and perceive the interconnectedness of everything in life. In addition, deep relaxation enables vital energy to circulate freely through the meridian pathways, which is essential for emotional healing.

Now that you have an understanding of how deep breathing and relaxation enhance acupressure for emotional balancing, you are ready to apply acupressure for specific common emotional complaints.

Hands-On Diary

There are many benefits of keeping a personal account of the changes that occur as you use acupressure. Although acupressure can produce immediate relief from stress and traumatic experiences, sometimes weeks may pass before you notice major changes in how you feel and in your ability to deal with your personal issues. Using this Hands-On Diary to record your week-by-week progress can heighten your awareness of how the techniques have facilitated your emotional healing. Making the extra effort to write down what points you used and how you felt later can enable you to know clearly how your body responds and thus what is most effective for your well-being.

HANDS-ON DIARY

Keeping Track of Your Self-Care Acupressure Practice

I am dealing with the following:
- ❑ Emotions _____
- ❑ Stress in my life _____
- ❑ Ailments _____
- ❑ Other _____

I have been practicing the self-acupressure instructions in:

Chapter _____, called _____, on pages ___–___

Chapter _____, called _____, on pages ___–___

I practice these exercises ❑ 10 ❑ 20 ❑ 30 ❑ 45 ❑ 60 minutes a day.

Mark the drawings to the right in red ink where you feel discomfort; mark the points you have used in blue ink.

The following seem to make my problem(s) worse:
- ❑ Stress
- ❑ Lack of exercise
- ❑ Constipation
- ❑ Emotional upset
- ❑ Menstruation
- ❑ Others _____

Describe the changes you noticed during the first three days of doing your routine:

_____

_____

_____

Describe the changes you felt after one full week of self-acupressure:

_____

_____

Describe the changes you noticed in your overall feeling of well-being after two or three weeks of doing self-acupressure:

_____

_____

5

ABANDONMENT

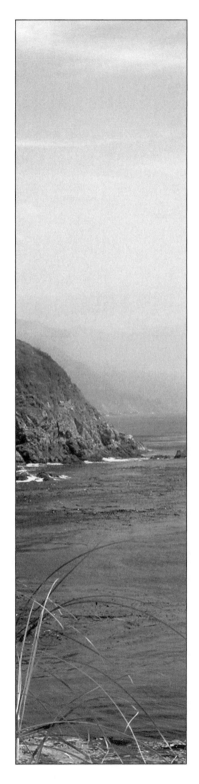

A bandonment by a parent or other important person during childhood can be traumatic. It leaves us with the sense that the people meant to care for us will fail to provide the emotional support we need, because they are unstable or will leave us. We may go through life trying to avoid feeling abandoned again. We hang on because being in an abusive relationship is better than being left alone—our greatest fear.

Many things may lead to a sense of abandonment:

- The arrival of a new sibling, or illness in an existing sibling, causing a loss of attention

- A parent who left through divorce or death

- A parent who was a substance abuser, was depressed or mentally ill, or worked long hours or at a distance

- A family that was frequently separated

- Warring parents who made the environment seem unstable or as if the family would break up

- Parents who overprotected their children, causing them to greatly fear handling life alone

- Being sent to a boarding school, institution, orphanage, or foster home

Becky's chronic depression, stomach pain, and cocaine addiction stemmed from being abandoned as a child. When she was eight years old, her parents divorced. Secrecy was the worst part of the divorce; her parents never talked, fought, or showed any feelings. Becky had no idea the divorce was even coming, or that her mother was having a secret affair with Becky's father's best friend. One minute everything was picture perfect, the next minute her whole world turned upside down.

Abandonment threatens our survival. It makes us feel unwanted, and we doubt our right to be here. It elicits fear, which may inhibit appropriate responses to common situations. For instance, if we fear abandonment as adults, we may be afraid to speak up in our relationships about the things we do not like for fear of being abandoned again. Or we may accept abandonment too readily, and interpret the slightest criticism or mood change from our partner as a signal that we are unwanted.

— Anodea Judith
Eastern Body Western Mind

Becky's father was the person she loved most in life. His attention and love made her feel special and important. Without warning or explanation, in reaction to the traumatic affair by Becky's mother, he moved out of state and cut off all communication. This trauma created an open wound that affected Becky for years.

Like many children of divorce, Becky blamed herself; she felt helpless and depressed. Many preteens experiment with drugs, alcohol, and sex. A long-term effect of divorce on girls, some experts say, is a greater likelihood of divorce themselves. All of these statistics held true for Becky.

Creating drama and chaos became her way of getting the attention and love she needed to cope with her deep feelings of abandonment. She continually relived the emotional pain of losing her father in other relationships. At thirteen her drug, alcohol, and sexual experimentation began. She was placed in foster care several times due to her mother's instability. At fifteen she dropped out of high school, moved in with an aunt, and had the first of her four children. She went from relationship to relationship, hoping to fill the void she had felt when she lost her father.

Parents and caregivers create the foundation for a child's self-image and future relationships. If a family does not express affection and the parents are unresponsive, other dysfunctional relationships can occur. An emotionally neglected child may seek attention from a teacher at school or another adult. When a child does not receive the love and attention he or she needs, a repetitious cycle of unmet emotional needs and distrust can be established. This in turn can cause emotional obsessions and unhealthy drives.

A child's primary relationships thus play a vital role in providing a foundation of trust. When a significant relationship ends suddenly without warning, the abandoned person can experience emotional shock. Psychological damage can occur due to death, divorce, physical abuse, or chemical dependency. Abandonment and betrayal make a person question their ability to love or be loved.

By the age of twenty-two, Becky had already been married and divorced twice. Her history of abusive relationships accentuated her deep longing for stability and love. After years of being estranged, time began to heal the distance between Becky and her mother. Her mother's life had turned in a new direction through a recovery process that included counseling, massage, antidepressant medication, and acupressure therapy. When Becky began to share with her mother that she suffered with painful stomachaches and feelings of abandonment, her mother was eager to suggest acupressure sessions for her.

Acupressure for Abandonment

Acupressure therapy can safely release traumatic experiences. Acupressure points are key areas that store painful emotions and events; holding these points causes deep muscular tension to relax, increasing circulation, heightening body awareness, and allowing old memories to surface. Strengthening your will can heal abandonment issues and dysfunctional patterns.

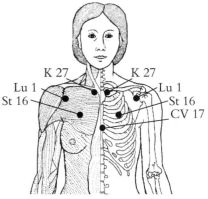

Becky's acupressure sessions transformed her negative emotions and stomach pain. Holding the upper chest points Lu 1 and K 27 got her in touch with her feelings of emptiness and anxiety. Holding points in the diaphragm resolved her stomach pain by releasing old anger and memories stored from childhood. Becky experienced a natural high by repeatedly holding St 16 and CV 17. This heightened sense of awareness nourished her spirit and motivated her to create a healthier life.

Within a month Becky was actively involved in her own recovery. She attended a weekly support group and a spiritual group that her mother utilized, she did daily self-acupressure, and she had weekly appointments with a chemical dependency counselor. She attended weekly acupressure sessions with her acupressure therapist and was encouraged to explore a "rebuilding diet," which included commonsense meals with a focus on additional vegetables and quality proteins. (See Chapter 26.) Meditation, affirmations, and point routines healed her wounded heart and paved the way for emotional vitality and balance. Two years later Becky was happily remarried and had successfully recreated her vision of family.

No matter how hard an abandoned person tries to fill their emptiness—through self-medication, drugs, alcohol, excessive food, or sex—self-destructive patterns continue. Connecting with the deep roots of your emotional pain is necessary for your recovery and healing. Dealing with each layer is imperative.

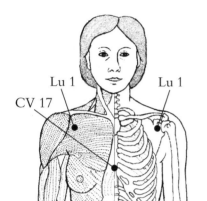

The following self-acupressure routines—along with wise life choices, emotional support, and perseverance—can break dysfunctional cycles.

Abandonment Meditation

Sit comfortably on a mat, blanket, or in a chair. Gently massage your neck, arms, shoulders, hands, torso, legs, and feet. Breathe deeply into your body as you release any stress and tension for two minutes. Close your eyes, and take slow, deep breaths. Drop your shoulders, straighten your spine, and place your hands on CV 17 at the center of your breastbone. Allow yourself to go back to the root experiences in your life where you felt abandoned while breathing deeply.

As you continue to hold CV 17, explore for at least a couple minutes how being abandoned stole your power and prevented you from living to the fullest… Search your mind for images,

Affirmations to Counteract Abandonment

- *I trust myself and will not abandon the love inside my heart.*

- *I am being taken care of by the universe.*

- *I am capable and lovable just as I am.*

- *Through deep breathing, I let go of hurtful relationships.*

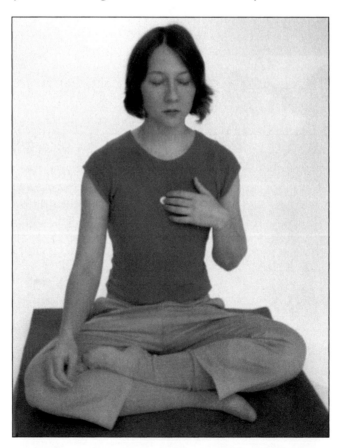

memories, and faces of the people who hurt you... Breathe deeply, and release any negative thoughts... Continue for three minutes.

Now cross your arms over your breastbone, placing your hands onto the upper, outer chest on Lu 1. Feel the warmth of your hug. Appreciate yourself for what you've just experienced. Breathe deeply into your heart, and affirm your place in the universe. Slowly release your pressure, allowing your hands to glide gently into your lap. Stretch your arms, rotate your wrists, and slowly open your eyes. Sit quietly for an additional minute to reflect on your experience and discover the benefits.

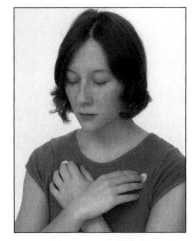

QUICK TIPS FOR ABANDONMENT

Use any of these self-care techniques to calm yourself when feelings of abandonment are triggered.

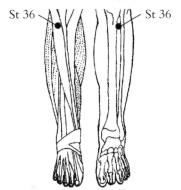

Deep Breathing: Do long, slow, deep breathing for five minutes. Imagine that each exhalation is a vehicle for releasing emotionally charged memories. Breathing slowly and deeply enables your body to assimilate greater amounts of oxygen, which has a calming effect when you feel anxious or abandoned.

Foot & Hand Massage: Sit comfortably and massage your feet and hands thoroughly for several minutes. Spend time on each finger and toe. Then, as you breathe deeply into your belly, rotate your wrists and ankles. This self-massage refocuses your mind on the present moment, instead of being scattered or drained by an abandonment issue.

Briskly Rub St 36: Use your fists to rub over St 36 (on the outside of the shinbones, below your knees) for one minute. This is a key point for heightening body awareness, emotional stamina, and inner strength. It also brings your attention out of the past and into the present moment. Use St 36 whenever you feel abandoned and an emotional outbreak occurs unexpectedly.

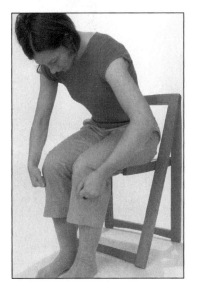

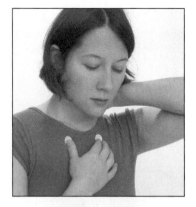

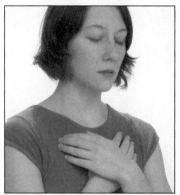

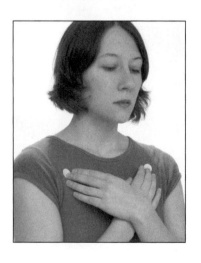

Neck Massage with K 27: Use one hand to knead and squeeze your neck muscles. Use your other hand to hold both K 27 points (below the inside edge of the collarbone, in the hollow spaces). Breathe deeply into your heart to calm yourself, and let go of any negative emotions and feelings of insecurity. Massaging your neck at K 27 can open your throat, free your voice, and empower you to express your feelings.

Palm CV 17: With your eyes closed, palm CV 17. Focus on breathing deeply for three minutes, keeping your spine straight. Before opening your eyes, slowly let your hands float down into your lap. To balance your emotions when an abandonment issue surfaces, lightly touch your thumb and middle finger together on each hand while breathing deeply.

SELF-CARE ROUTINE FOR ABANDONMENT

Make yourself comfortable sitting in a chair for the following acupressure routine.

Step 1

Hold Lu 1: As you breathe deeply into your body, hold Lu 1 (which is on the outer portion of your chest, four finger-widths up from the armpit crease and one finger-width inward) for two minutes. Notice any body sensations, and breathe deeply, paying attention to any emotions that surface. Abandonment is often layered with underlying anger, sadness, fear, and resentment. Allow plenty of time to feel these emotions. Focus on the images connected to what you are feeling. Allow yourself to make sounds, and let your feelings out to express yourself. If you are uncomfortable making sounds, concentrate on making each breath slow and deep.

Step 2

Hold St 16: Place your hands on both sides of the upper chest to hold St 16 (above the center of the breastbone, in the indentation between the ribs). Breathe deeply as you thank yourself for having the courage to face the unknown. Take a moment to appreciate how your body has protected you, and breathe into your heart.

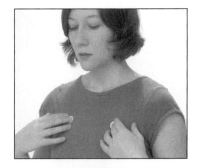

Step 3

Hold Sp 16: Hold Sp 16 (located underneath the lower edge of the ribcage, a half-inch in from the nipple line). Breathe into your belly for two minutes. Focus on letting go of any emotional charge with each complete exhalation, blowing out any negative feelings or images linked with being abandoned in your life.

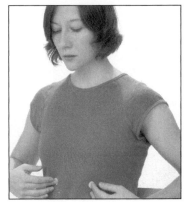

Step 4

Palm CV 17: Palm CV 17 (in the center of your breastbone). Inhale deeply as you turn your head slowly to the left, focusing on any negative images or tensions you may have. Exhale as you slowly turn your head to the right, releasing these memories and tensions. Continue for two minutes, consciously letting go of any distress. Continue longer if you feel unfinished.

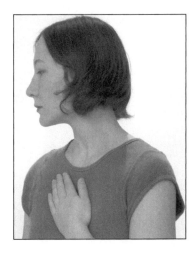

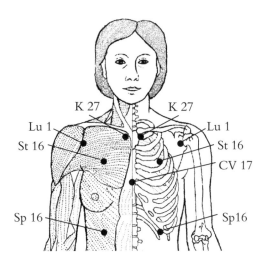

Trying to love another when you do not love yourself does not work. You end up feeling possessive, jealous, and dependent. By contrast, when you really begin to love yourself, you become a magnet, attracting the love of others.

— Margo Anand
The Erotic Impulse

Step 5

Rest & Reflection: Cover yourself with a light blanket, and allow yourself to rest with your eyes closed for five minutes. Afterward spend ten minutes writing down your feelings and experiences.

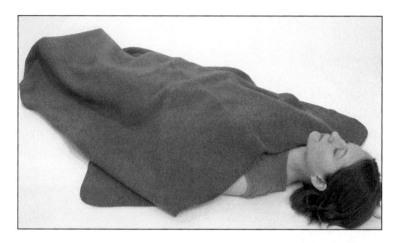

Remember to rest after acupressure; releasing your feelings can be exhausting. Without deep relaxation, toxic emotions released from the musculature can get blocked. Five to ten minutes of complete relaxation along with deep breathing is an essential part of acupressure's emotional balancing process. Resolving abandonment issues takes patience, time, support, and self-love.

6

ADDICTION

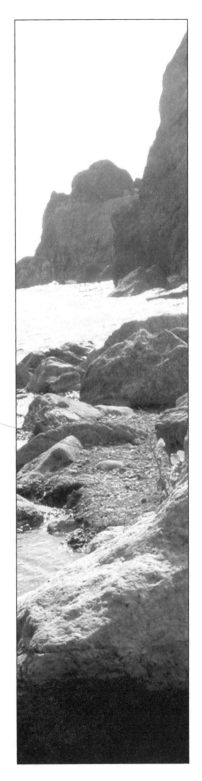

There are many types and degrees of addiction, ranging from mild habitual lifestyle patterns to severe drug abuse. Although our focus here is on common repetitive negative behaviors and bad habits such as eating disorders, gambling, and smoking, people with more serious addictions such as alcohol or drug abuse can also benefit from regularly practicing the routines in this chapter.

To overcome an addiction using acupressure, a person must first want to change and be willing to make an effort to stop the addictive cycle. Some acupressure points can strengthen a person's willpower; but we also recommend getting guidance from a counselor, therapist, or community support group, such as a twelve-step program.

Dependency, insecurity, or an emotional wound can create enough emptiness and desire to drive a person into an addiction, resulting in an uncontrollable urge. Fulfilling this craving by consuming a substance (be it alcohol, cocaine, caffeine, or nicotine) or by exhibiting a problem behavior (involving gambling, sex, eating, or spending) may at first seem to fill that hole, but it actually further reinforces the dependency. An unhealthy habit that is out of control can sabotage a relationship and cause you to make poor decisions that limit your personal growth and ruin the quality of your life.

Whether the substance abuse is focused on drugs, alcohol, tobacco, or food, the addiction—which begins as a way of escaping or easing pain—affects the brain. When acupressure points are pressed steadily for at least one minute, neurochemicals called endorphins change the brain chemistry, which affects the perceptions related to addiction and rebalances the body's metabolism. For this reason, acupuncture, which uses the same points as acupressure, is particularly effective with drug abuse and smoking cessation in easing the negative side effects of quitting. Although

Affirmations to Counteract Addictions

- *I trust myself to make wise decisions.*

- *I love myself for all I have gone through.*

- *I release my guilt and let go of any regret.*

- *I vow to take care of myself in a good way.*

- *I am a child of the universe and am grateful for what I have.*

- *I am responsible and capable of living a great life.*

scientists have made great strides in understanding how addictive substances work on the brain, they haven't figured out the exact causes of alcohol and drug dependency and abuse. Years of research point toward some inheritable or biological factors; psychological and social factors aren't entirely understood, but they play an important role as well.

Adolescents and adults are most at risk for addictive behavior when their need for love, approval, and validation—the unconditional love that every newborn and young child needs and has a right to—goes unmet during childhood. If you have been mistreated most of your life, it's hard to treat yourself well. Destructive role models can damage your self-image. Having unreliable parents who are unable to meet your needs can affect your self-esteem and how you take care of yourself.

The unconscious nature of addictions is what makes solving them so difficult. Some substance abusers recognize that they have a serious, out-of-control problem; others, for whatever reason, seem unable to face up to their addictions. Addictive cycles are cumulative; one stress leads to another. For example, making poor choices and putting oneself into emotionally unhealthy situations lead to muscular tensions, pressures, and pain. Drugs, alcohol, or cigarettes can dull the stress and tension temporarily, so the cycle continues.

The physical touch of acupressure, which releases pain, mental stress, and physical tension while heightening awareness, can support you in breaking the cycle of addiction. Certain acupressure points, when pressed, cause an endorphin release, and help you relax and regain the willpower and intention to move in a new direction. There are acupressure points for regaining stability, reducing cravings, and heightening morale, self-esteem, and self-confidence—all of which are vital for combating addictions.

In contrast to the numbing effects of drugs, holding acupressure points increases circulation, returning the person to the present moment. By "lifting the fog" of addiction and becoming aware of your patterns, you can begin to make conscious efforts to change those patterns. That means choosing to be around people and do activities that will support your efforts to fight your addictions.

Alice lived in an abusive marriage with her alcoholic husband and their three children. Her life was tough, but alcohol, cigarettes, and gambling took the edge off and helped her cope emotionally with her lousy relationship and difficult kids. She worked full time as a maintenance person in a department store, where she did hard, physically demanding labor. Her children were always in trouble at school because of the neglect and mistreatment they received at home.

Alice's parents were alcoholic and abusive, making them unpredictable and emotionally unreliable. Their neglect forced Alice to become responsible at a young age for adult tasks. Overwhelmed and out of her league, she began a cycle of self-destructive behaviors, using alcohol, smoking cigarettes, and getting into unhealthy relationships. Just as Alice's parents had failed to support her, she failed to love and esteem herself and her own children. Patterns set in motion by parents tend to be repeated and passed from one generation to the next: neither Alice nor her husband had learned the necessary parental skills of expressing unconditional love and setting healthy limits.

When she was only forty years old, Alice was in emotional pain and very poor health. She suffered from stress-related digestive disorders and fibromyalgia, a chronic neuromuscular condition that made her muscles and back hurt most of the time. Doctors were unable to help her. Her pain became so unbearable that she decided to look into alternative health care. She was referred to Beth Henning, who over time was able to help her break the cycle. Instead of resorting to back surgery, she used self-acupressure, breathing exercises, and positive visualizations to empower her life.

During her first acupressure sessions, Alice's back pain remained constant. Since the acupressure touch brought attention to her body, she became more acutely aware of the pain. The first three weeks were the most difficult: the pain taxed her energy, making her feel more depressed. Her breakthrough came when her emotions began to surface and she was able to release some of her pent-up anguish and despair. Acupressure thus released her emotional and physical pain and enabled her to get closer to the core of her healing. After four months of weekly sessions with Beth, Alice was able to use self-acupressure on her own, which provided a way for her to become self-reliant instead of self-

In our daily life problems invariably arise. But problems themselves do not automatically cause suffering. If we can directly address our problem and focus our energies on finding a solution, for instance, the problem can be transformed into a challenge. If we throw into the mix, however, a feeling that our problem is "unfair," we add an additional ingredient that can become a powerful fuel in creating mental unrest and emotional suffering.

— His Holiness
the Dalai Lama
The Art of Happiness

When you forgive yourself, self-acceptance begins and self-love grows. That is the supreme forgiveness—when you finally forgive yourself.

— Don Miguel Ruiz
The Mastery of Love

destructive. The support she got from Beth's acupressure sessions, and her strong desire to heal, empowered her to curtail her addictions, get out of her abusive marriage, and be more present for her children.

Food & Sugar Addictions

A common form of addiction involves eating. How you eat often reflects your self-image and your feelings. For instance, when you feel depressed or unworthy, food cravings and overeating can fill you up—literally—masking emotional pain. Food addictions are also common when stress levels are high. Acupressure is effective for balancing the metabolism and reducing the stress that commonly drives people to compulsive eating disorders.

Food is a basic need, providing nutrients and sensual pleasure, but eating addictive foods creates a vicious cycle. Foods containing sugar, yeast, and alcohol feed the detrimental yeast in your body and can trigger emotional instability and upheaval. The more this type of yeast grows, the more your body craves sugar, creating a condition known as Candida or a yeast infection. The remedy is to starve the bacteria feeding on the sugar. Work toward the goal of eliminating all sweets such as sugar, honey, corn syrup, and cane juice. In addition, cut out alcohol and even fruit except for a small amount of apples or pears. This dietary practice, if strictly followed for four to six months, can break a sugar addiction.

Most people feel they cannot completely eliminate addictive foods, but avoiding them can be challenging and takes discipline. You can use it as an opportunity to grow stronger physically and psychologically. Use your willpower and intention to break the cycle; by ending your addiction to sweets, you become empowered and gain self-confidence. You will find several ways to overcome food and sugar addictions in the following exercises and routines.

QUICK TIPS FOR ADDICTION

Practice any of these acupressure techniques to break addictive patterns:

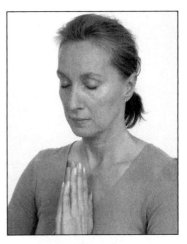

Breathe into CV 17: Bring the palms of your hands together at the center of your chest. Using the side of your thumb knuckle, press the Sea of Tranquility point (CV 17, on the center of your breastbone). Breathe slowly and deeply into your heart for two minutes to calm yourself, reduce stress, and balance your emotions.

Hold the Temples & Chew: Place your fingertips on your temples, in the hollow areas level with and just outside your eyebrows. Place your thumbs between your upper and lower jaws and press the muscle that pops out when you chew. Clench your back teeth as if you were chewing, then release. Clench and release in a rhythmic pattern, approximately once per second. Each time you clench down on your molars, you should also feel a muscle pop out in the temple area underneath your fingertips. Exerting steady finger pressure on these points with the muscle movement, coupled with long, deep breathing, will activate areas of the brain that govern addictions and obsessions as well as TMJ jaw problems. If you find holding your arms up to be difficult, rest your elbows on a table; do as much as you can, and build up your timing slowly on your own.

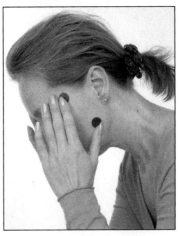

Upper Chest Press (St 16): Place your fingertips into the hollows directly above the breast tissue between the third and fourth ribs. Close your eyes for one minute as you breathe deeply to let go of any addictive desires or negative thoughts.

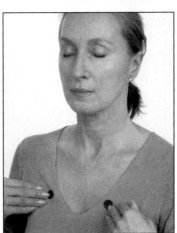

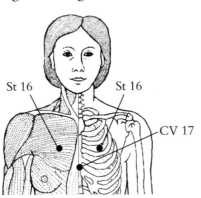

St 16   St 16

CV 17

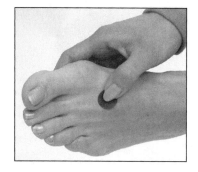

Massage & Hold Feet (Lv 3): Slowly knead both feet for one minute. Grasp the webbing between the large and index toes to hold Lv 3 with firm steady pressure. Breathe deeply into your belly for an additional minute to balance addictive cravings.

NATURAL HIGH SELF-CARE ROUTINE

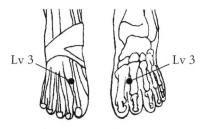

Lv 3   Lv 3

Sit comfortably in a chair. This five-minute self-acupressure routine uses special points that release endorphins, the neurochemicals that have a euphoric effect. The more regularly you practice this routine, the better the results.

Step 1

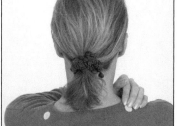

Shoulder Massage (GB 21, TW 15): Slowly and thoroughly knead your shoulder muscles, applying and releasing pressure for three to five seconds at a time. Continue massaging this area rhythmically with your eyes closed for at least one minute.

Step 2

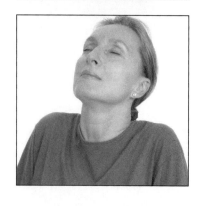

Shoulder Shrug: Sit on the edge of your chair with your spine straight, and place your hands on your knees. Inhale deeply as you shrug your shoulders up toward your earlobes. Hold the breath for two seconds. Exhale as you drop your shoulders downward. Continue for one minute while you breathe deeply through the nose, if possible. If breathing through your nose is difficult or impossible, create a small opening with your mouth, as if you were sipping a straw. Breathing in this manner or through your nose will help prevent hyperventilation. On the last shoulder shrug, inhale and hold your breath for ten seconds. Exhale slowly and smoothly as you let your shoulders relax downward.

Step 3

Gates of Consciousness Press (GB 20): Place your thumbs underneath the base of the skull, about three inches apart; feel for a hollow area under the bone structure. Slowly tilt your head back as you apply steady pressure underneath the skull. Close your eyes and begin long, deep breathing, maintaining firm pressure for one minute. Let your hands float down into your lap, and gently shake your shoulders to relax. Holding the Gates of Consciousness points can increase your awareness and help you to make wiser decisions.

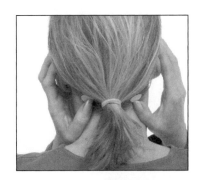

Step 4

Top of Head & Base of Spine (GV 20, GV 1): Curve the fingertips of your right hand, and place them gently on the top, center of your head. Place your left hand at the base of your tailbone and press upward. Breathe deeply for one minute with your eyes closed. Feel or imagine the connection between the points and the energy circulating through your spine. This point combination releases endorphins, the neurochemicals that produce a natural high.

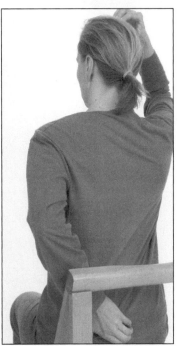

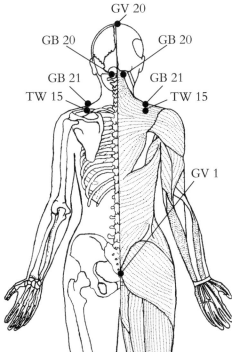

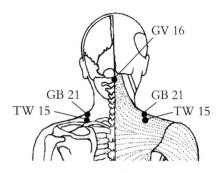

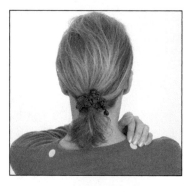

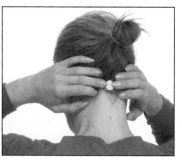

Step 5

Foot & Ankle Massage (Lv 3, Sp 3, K 6): Slowly knead and squeeze your right foot and ankle as you breathe deeply into your belly for one minute. Then knead and squeeze your left foot and ankle. Now rotate your ankles and wrists ten times in each direction simultaneously. Finish by gently stretching any tension out of your body.

SELF-CARE ROUTINE FOR ADDICTION

The following self-care routine begins by working on the shoulders. Chronic tension in the shoulders creates tightness and irritability; both can inhibit good judgment. The routine then uses points under the base of the skull and on the head to rebalance areas related to stress. Practice this routine two times a day to strengthen your willpower to fight against addictions.

Find a quiet, private place to practice, sitting comfortably in a chair with your spine straight.

Step 1

Shoulder Massage (GB 21, TW 15): Knead your shoulders firmly in slow motion as you breathe deeply for one minute.

Step 2

Center Base of Skull Press (GV 16): Place your middle fingers in the large hollow at the center of the base of your skull. Gradually press for one minute with your head tilted back slightly. Concentrate on taking long, deep breaths.

Step 3

Gentle Forehead Touch (GB 14): Place your middle fingertips on both sides of your forehead, one finger-width above the eyebrow in line with the center of the eye. Breathe slowly and deeply with your eyes closed while lightly touching GB 14 for at least a minute. This point clears the mind, balances the emotions, releases mental distress, and transforms the self-sabotaging nature of addictions.

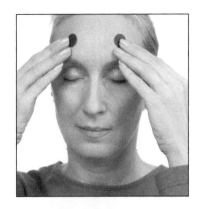

Step 4

Base of Ribs Press (Sp 16): Place your fingertips on the base of your ribcage into all the rib notches with your fingers curved. Rub along the base of the rib to feel for indentations in the bone structure. Place your fingertips in these notches while you breathe long and deep for one minute. This practice strengthens your self-image and releases tension in the diaphragm.

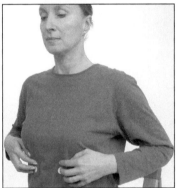

Step 5

Center of Stomach Press (CV 12, CV 14):★ Place your fingertips three to four finger-widths above your navel in your stomach area, directly below the center of your breastbone. Take slow, deep breaths while you hold these upper abdominal points for one minute. This pressure will release emotional stress stored in the stomach, balance your sense of personal power, and release the tensions associated with negative compulsions.

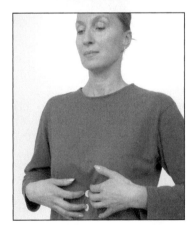

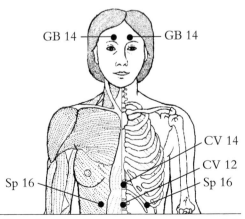

★Do not press these points if you have an ulcer or hernia, your stomach is full, or you are using medications.

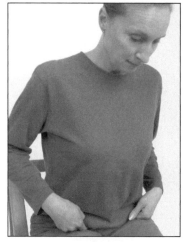

Step 6

Rushing Doors (Sp 12, Sp 13): Place your fingertips in your groin, midway between the outer tip of your pubic bone and your hipbone. Feel for the cordlike ligament in this area. With your fingers curved, gradually apply firm pressure on this ligament as you breathe deeply into your belly for one minute. Releasing these points can bring deep relaxation and renew your sense of self.

Step 7

Final Balancing (GV 24.5, CV 17): Place the middle finger of your left hand lightly between your eyebrows (GV 24.5), where the bridge of the nose meets the bottom of your forehead. Place the fingers of your right hand firmly into the hollows at the center of your breastbone (CV 17). Consciously breathe slowly and deeply, placing your attention on the forehead points for one minute to balance your emotions, increase your morale, and further develop your spiritual awareness.

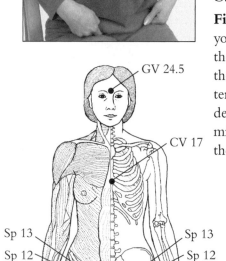

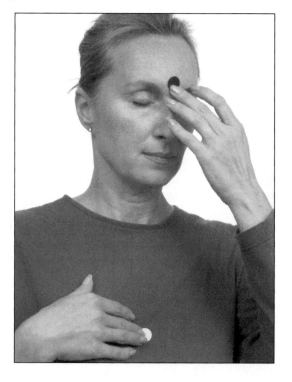

7

ANGER

We know that when angry feelings arise, the adrenal glands produce stress hormones in response to signals from the brain. Stress hormones speed up the heart rate, sending energy rushing to muscles and other organs, inhibiting some bodily functions like digestion. Anger can constrict the blood vessels to the digestive tract, taxing the cardiovascular system and causing hypertension, insomnia, and headaches.

Acupressure releases muscular tension that can result from harboring anger. Unexpressed anger stored in the body commonly accumulates in the shoulders, neck, and jaw muscles and also in the mid- to upper back region and pelvis. Holding acupressure points in these areas can enable the causes of anger to surface and release unresolved issues.

Anger is commonly thought of as being a negative, destructive emotion that can rage out of control. Certainly over time it can become highly self-destructive and harmful to your health and mental well-being. Constant exposure to stress hormones may impair the immune system and other functions. But anger is not always bad; when it is expressed and balanced, this powerful emotion can be used productively as a driving force for motivation and fueling creativity.

Anger produces the chemical ingredients necessary for you to have the inner strength to stand up for what you know is right. You can then consciously use your anger in an empowering way to assert yourself. Once your anger has been expressed constructively and released, you are free to engage creatively and make new choices in your life. Using deep breathing and emotional balancing points specific to anger will allow your body's energy to flow more freely. Deep breathing, along with the ancient healing art of acupressure, will increase the circulation of nutrients to the cells of your body, heightening your energy and emotional

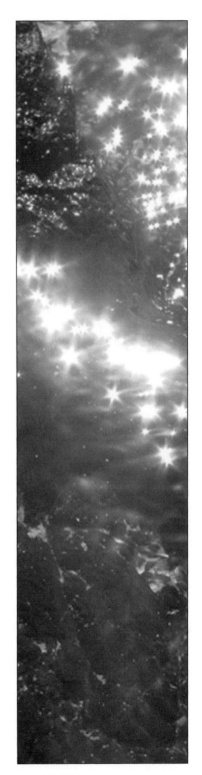

Affirmations to Counteract Anger

- *As I breathe deeply, I am transforming my frustration and anger into positive energy.*

- *I am using my anger to propel my personal growth and goals.*

- *I am assertive in a healthy way.*

- *I release and I let go.*

- *I speak my truth with grace.*

awareness. This will enable you to be more stable as you experience your anger. When you are feeling secure and breathing deeply, you are able to see more of your options and make productive, empowering choices.

When anger is released by holding acupressure points and breathing deeply, healthier chemical patterns are restored and your muscles relax. Breathing deeply and consciously releasing your anger helps counteract the physiological stress that this emotion produces in your body. In addition, acupressure opens your breathing passages, enabling you to receive more oxygen.

Don, a middle-aged businessman, was in turmoil with himself and his family over various issues. He resented his older brother for overpowering him. His wife had recently discovered her past sexual abuse and was projecting fear, betrayal, and insecurity onto their relationship. Their four children were acting out through drugs, sex, and skipping school. As a result, Don was depressed, angry, and in an emotional crisis.

Don also had a range of physical problems. He had ulcer pain, shoulder and neck tension, jaw pain, headaches, and a history of unstable blood pressure. His family doctor had prescribed a variety of medications, including antidepressants. The medications didn't help his physical pain and made him numb emotionally. He turned to alcohol to drown out his pain.

Don decided to pursue acupressure as an alternative therapy. His acupressure sessions always included a shoulder and neck release. He soon learned this shoulder and neck point routine to practice on himself at home. His chronic shoulder and neck tensions released as he vented his rage about his wife's projections. Releasing his frustration enabled him to express his anger and other feelings in a much more productive way; he was also able to be more supportive and patient with his wife as she went through therapy.

Through acupressure, Don discovered that the anger stuck in his gut was causing his ulcer and headache pain. Once the points in this area were released, these physical symptoms and the depression went away. Learning and applying proper food combinations and self-acupressure techniques helped Don's digestive and stress-related problems.

In addition to self-acupressure, Don began a regular exercise program to routinely release his stored-up tension. He also spent fifteen minutes a day in meditation and prayer. He found the wisdom to let go of the situations and people he could not control. Within one month Don's physical symptoms diminished, his family relationships with his children improved remarkably, and he no longer felt on edge with his older brother.

Common Symptoms of Suppressed Anger

Any of the following physical symptoms can occur when anger becomes blocked inside of the body:

- chronic shoulder tension
- teeth grinding
- neck tension and headaches
- exhaustion
- heart disease or stroke
- insomnia
- high blood pressure
- digestive problems

Survivors of Abuse

Anger is a natural response when a person's integrity is violated. In order to deal with daily life, victims of abuse often block their emotions and dissociate from the pain. Unfortunately, suppressed anger leads to depression. Many survivors of abuse have found that releasing their anger directly at their violators is healing and empowering. With the emotional support of a psychotherapist, they can do this by visualizing their violator's presence. Once the anger begins to release, the dark cloud of depression and sadness lifts, and situations in life become clearer.

Positive Lifestyle Considerations

Traditional Chinese medicine teaches the following lifestyle changes for balancing anger.

- **Stretch Several Times a Day:** Stretching your body regularly is the most important activity you can do to balance your anger. The more you develop flexibility through stretching, the more you'll be able to channel your anger in constructive, creative ways.

You must forgive those who hurt you, even if whatever they did to you is unforgivable in your mind. You will forgive them not because they deserve to be forgiven, but because you don't want to suffer and hurt yourself every time you remember what they did to you.

— Don Miguel Ruiz
The Mastery of Love

- **Practice Co-Counseling:** Joining a co-counseling group is a safe, inexpensive way to process and release your anger and resentment. (See Appendix D for more information.)

- **Eat Plenty of Green Vegetables:** Eat them lightly steamed or raw. The minerals, vitamins, chlorophyll, and life energy contained in green vegetables can balance anger.

- **Consciously Reduce the Amount of Oil:** Avoid eating fried foods such as potato chips, French fries, fried chicken, and other fast foods. Excessive oil taxes the liver and affects how you deal with your anger.

- **Avoid Eating Sugar:** This will stabilize your system and emotions and decrease mood swings.

- **Eat Sour Foods:** such as lemon juice or sauerkraut in moderation. The sour taste helps to cleanse the liver and balance anger.

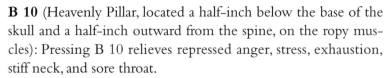

SPECIAL ACUPRESSURE POINTS FOR BALANCING ANGER

Once you practice these easy hands-on techniques and become familiar with them, teach them to your children or friends to enable them to manage anger, too.

GB 20 (Gates of Consciousness, located below the base of the skull, in the hollow between the two vertical neck muscles): Holding GB 20 relieves frustration, anger, headaches, mental stress, and arthritis in the shoulders and neck.

B 10 (Heavenly Pillar, located a half-inch below the base of the skull and a half-inch outward from the spine, on the ropy muscles): Pressing B 10 relieves repressed anger, stress, exhaustion, stiff neck, and sore throat.

GB 21 (Shoulder Well, located on the top of the shoulder, two finger-widths from the side of the neck): GB 21 relieves irritability, anger, shoulder tension, and poor circulation. On a pregnant woman, this point should be pressed lightly, using greater sensitivity.

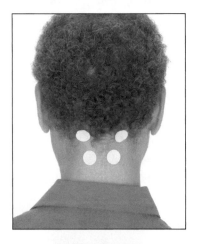

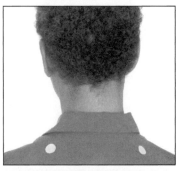

CV 12 (Center of Power, located on the center of the body, midway between the base of the breastbone and the belly button): Holding CV 12 relieves emotional stress, frustration, stomach pains, abdominal spasms, and headaches. Do not hold this point longer than two minutes, and do so only on an empty stomach.★

★*Caution:* Do not hold this point deeply if you have a serious illness such as heart disease, cancer, or high blood pressure.

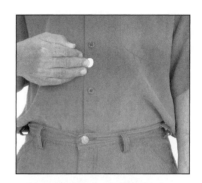

B 23, B 47 (Sea of Vitality, located between the second and third lumbar vertebrae, two to four finger-widths away from the spine, at waist level): Pressing B 23 and B 47 relieves depression, fatigue, exhaustion, trauma, anger, and fear.★

★*Caution:* Do not press on disintegrating disks or fractured or broken bones. If your back is in a weak condition, touch these points lightly, keeping your fingers stationary and exerting no pressure. See your doctor first if you have extreme back pain or need medical advice.

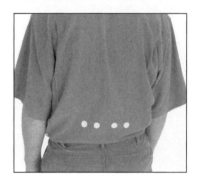

P 6 (Inner Gate, located in the middle of the inside of the forearm, three finger-widths from the wrist crease): Holding P 6 relieves excessive anger, shock, high fever, and exhaustion.

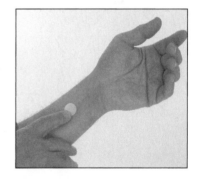

P 9 (Middle Rushing, located on the inside base of the nail of the middle finger): Holding P 9 relieves excessive anger, shock, high fever, and exhaustion. P 9 is traditionally used as an emergency revival point.

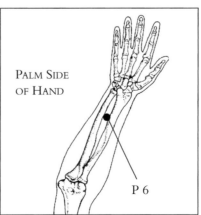

PALM SIDE OF HAND

P 6

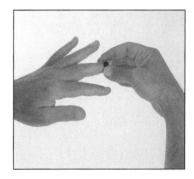

QUICK TIPS
FOR BALANCING ANGER

You may want to memorize and practice a few of the following techniques whenever you feel unwanted anger beginning to rise:

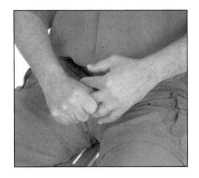

Hold the Middle Finger of Either Hand: Make a long *aaaaah* sound. Explore your feelings as you continue to make this sound and hold your middle finger for two minutes. If you are in a public place, making the sound is optional; you can simply exhale slowly through your mouth instead.

• **Drink Water When You Feel Angry:** Since anger has a fiery nature, drinking water can cool down your temper. Take slow, deep breaths as you sip a glass of cool water.

• **Inhale a Rose Smell or Rose Oil:** Doing so is deeply relaxing and balances anger. A rose's smell is associated with love and beauty.

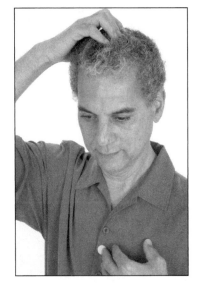

• **Work Hard & Exercise:** Performing hard physical work can be an excellent way to channel your anger. Next time you feel frustrated or angry, prepare a garden, dig a hole, or run up a hill. A regular exercise program, combining aerobics and stretching, helps to discharge anger. You can also use the first exercise in the next self-care routine, called Angry Eyes Punching Out, to release stored tension and frustration.

Do Shoulder Massage & Hold Emotional Balancing Points: Spend three minutes massaging your shoulders and neck while consciously focusing on your breath. Then place the fingertips of your right hand at GV 20 (on top of your head), while your left hand holds CV 17. Close your eyes, and breathe comfortably for two minutes. Affirm the following to yourself: "I am calm and centered in the midst of it all."

Use Fists at Diaphragm & Groin Points: Lie down comfortably on your stomach. Place the palms of your hands comfortably over the center of your belly, at CV 12.★ Breathe deeply into this key point for releasing anger and frustration. Next, place your fingertips or fists on Sp 12 and Sp 13 (in the groin, where your upper thighs meet the trunk of your body). Raise your head and feet in the air while breathing deeply for ten to twenty seconds. Then relax completely for two minutes.

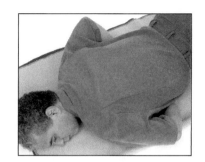

★*Caution:* Do not use CV 12 if you are pregnant or have a serious medical condition.

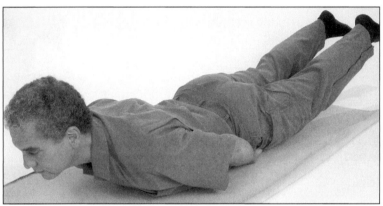

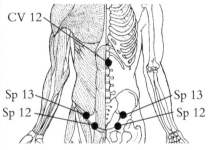

Do a Cross Hug: Cross your hands in front of you so your fingertips hold the center of the armpit on the opposite side. Breathe deeply into your heart. Explore what you are angry about or how you have been violated. Holding yourself in this way can bring you to the source of your anger and whatever sadness may be deep inside your heart.

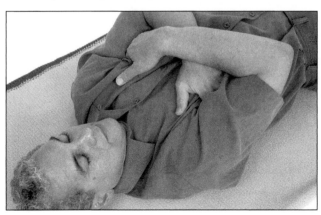

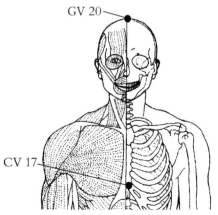

SELF-CARE ROUTINE
FOR BALANCING ANGER

Begin the following acupressure routine by standing comfortably.

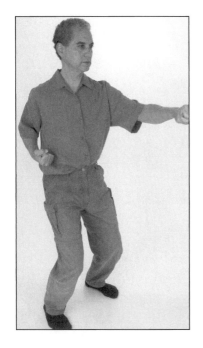

Step 1

Angry Eyes Punching Out: Stand with your feet comfortably apart and your knees bent slightly. Place your fists by your waist. Inhale, open your eyes wide, and clench your molars together firmly. Clench your fists and tighten your arm muscles as you exhale and slowly punch straight out in front of your body. Keeping your fists clenched, inhale as you slowly bring your fist back to the waist. Repeat the exercise two more times to each side. This exercise releases anger, frustration, irritation, resentment, and tension in the arms and chest. When practiced regularly it strengthens the vital organs and especially benefits the liver.

Sit comfortably for the remainder of this routine.

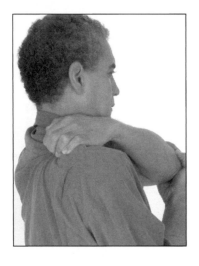

Step 2

Shoulder Grasp & Pull: Curve the fingers of your right hand over your left shoulder, hooking them onto the top of your shoulder muscle, close to the base of your neck. Inhale as you gradually apply firm pressure with your fingertips. Hold for a few seconds. Exhale slowly, raking your fingers over your shoulder, firmly stretching the muscle. Let your right hand fall back into your lap. Next, use your left hand to work on your right shoulder. Hook your fingers firmly into the muscle of your right shoulder. Inhale deeply as you apply firm, steady pressure with your fingers. Hold for a few seconds. Then exhale slowly, raking your fingers over your shoulder, giving a firm stretch to the muscle. Let your left hand float into your lap. Repeat the Shoulder Grasp & Pull for one minute, taking deep breaths.

Step 3

Shoulder Shrugs: Inhale deeply as you lift your shoulders up to your earlobes and tilt your head back. Exhale as you lower your head and your shoulders down and let yourself relax. Repeat this exercise for one minute, breathing as slowly and deeply as you can. This exercise releases the frustration, anger, and resentment stored in the shoulder muscles.

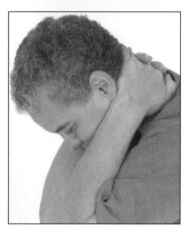

Step 4

Neck Press: Interlace your fingers together at the back of your neck and let your head hang forward, with your elbows close together and pointing down toward your lap. Inhale deeply, raising your head as you stretch your elbows out to the sides. Let your head tilt back. Exhale as your head relaxes forward and your elbows come close together in front of you. Repeat this exercise for one minute. Then let your hands float back into your lap and relax.

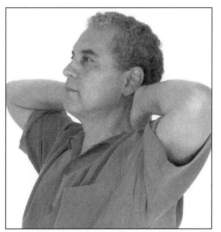

Step 5

Hold Your Middle Finger: Use your left hand to firmly grasp your right middle finger, resting your hands in your lap as you breathe deeply with your eyes closed for at least one minute. Then switch hands to hold the length of your left middle finger firmly. Take another minute with your eyes closed to breathe slowly and deeply. Holding the middle finger in this way stimulates acupressure points that release anger and resentment. You may find that holding your middle finger relieves anger as water puts out fire.

8

ANXIETY
& PANIC ATTACKS

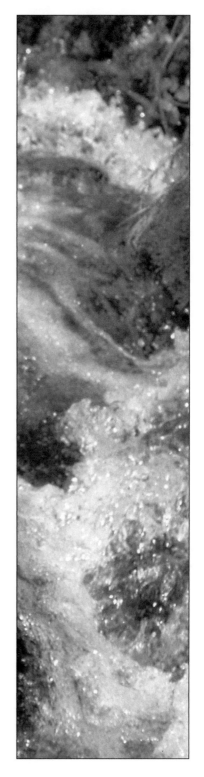

A nxiety is a normal human emotion, a reaction to an anticipated or imagined danger or event; fear, by contrast, involves a specific event and is a reaction to a perceived danger. We all feel anxious sometimes, from day-to-day pressures and stress to anticipating when something important is about to occur. Anxiety can motivate us to avoid danger or to work hard to achieve and be rewarded. But uncontrollable, extreme, or frequent anxiety can become harmful.

Highly anxious people experience excessive worry and tension much of the time; they rarely feel calm and relaxed. Anxiety can become a way of life, filled with muscle tension, headaches, gastrointestinal problems, aches and pains, insomnia, poor concentration, feeling restless or keyed up, irritability, or fatigue. Many people who suffer from anxiety seek help for their medical problems and don't realize that those troubles stem from an emotional imbalance.

The extreme anxiety of a panic attack is unpredictable and short-lived. Generally lasting ten to twenty minutes, a panic attack is characterized by a crescendo of fear, a suddenly accelerated heart rate, heart palpitations, difficulty breathing or shortness of breath, chest pain, shaking, sweating, and fear of losing control. A panic attack can be triggered by a memory of being threatened or abused; a buried traumatic experience can be the root cause.

Between panic attacks, emotional symptoms often persist. Some people become fearful that they'll have another attack, so they get anxious and worry. Phobias can develop when people go out of their way to avoid places and situations in which they had an attack.

Affirmations to Counteract Anxiety & Panic Attacks

- *I let go of my expectations.*

- *I trust that I will be taken care of.*

- *I am at peace with myself in the present moment.*

- *I consciously breathe deeply and let go of any anxiety.*

- *I am safe and let go of what the future may bring.*

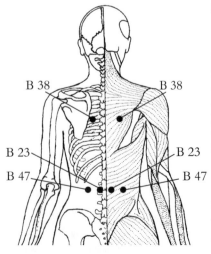

B 38   B 38

B 23   B 23

B 47   B 47

When Tony was seven years old, he was temporarily stuck in an elevator with his mother for one hour. Although many children who have similar experiences are not traumatized for life, Tony suffered from frequent nightmares, anxiety attacks, and interrupted sleep that affected his schoolwork. Tony's child psychologist recognized his symptoms as those of post-traumatic stress disorder and treated him with cognitive-behavioral therapy and diaphragmatic breathing. Cognitive-behavioral therapy, by coaching him to change his thoughts, taught him to react differently to feeling trapped.

Tony was the elder of two children, the center of attention until his sister Debbie was born two years before the elevator occurrence. He suffered intense sibling rivalry, which further contributed to his insecurity and anxiety. When he struggled to get attention through complaining, his sister would upstage him. His parents recognized the psychosomatic nature of their son's tummy aches and his inappropriate behavior in its early stages and provided him with excellent care. The cognitive-behavioral therapy stabilized his anxiety and the gastrointestinal problems he experienced during preadolescence. When his anxiety returned in his teenage years, Tony began seeing an adult psychotherapist.

Tony's psychotherapy sessions became more effective once he began receiving a series of weekly acupressure treatments as well. The deep relaxation from the acupressure supported his personal growth and motivated him to learn self-care to further relieve his stress and anxiety. Self-acupressure made him feel more self-reliant and confident. Psychotherapy and acupressure ultimately resolved his childhood trauma and eliminated his anxiety.

Acupressure relieves anxiety and panic attacks by releasing muscular tension. When acupressure points are held, life energy flows through the body, balancing the metabolism and calming the spirit. Free of tension, your breathing naturally deepens. This helps you to relax and to feel calmer and better about yourself. Deep relaxation can increase your awareness and provide new insights into issues affecting your anxiety. Acupressure therapy is an excellent adjunct to psychotherapy as well as medication, increasing the effectiveness of both approaches. Thus, we recommend a good course of acupressure, deep breathing, a balanced whole foods diet, and daily aerobic exercise in conjunction with these Western therapeutic treatments.

Road Anxiety

Meredith, an intelligent, healthy, middle-aged counselor, asked Michael Gach to help relieve her road anxiety. "I recently moved to a beautiful house in the countryside. I get the greatest anxiety attacks when I'm driving at speeds over forty-five miles per hour on highways and freeways. I'm okay driving slowly, but once I accelerate, I go into extreme panic and feel the need to use a restroom. Since I moved to the countryside, I am not familiar with places that offer a clean bathroom."

After explaining how acupressure works, Michael had Meredith lie down comfortably on her back. He started with points on her chest (Lu 1) to open up her breathing. As he held her lower back points (B 23, B 47) and the points between her shoulder blades (B 38), he encouraged her to relax and breathe deeply into her belly.

While Michael held her acupressure points, she breathed deeply and recalled some of her scary childhood experiences. Her forehead furrowed, remembering how frustrated and impatient her parents had been. He guided her to recollect driving with her parents. She remembered how out of control her father was on the freeway—a typical show-off middle-aged male driver who wouldn't stop the car for anything or anyone's urgent needs. Her eyes rolled back as she relived her panic and desperate need to go to the bathroom. No one in her family would listen to her. Meredith ended up wetting her pants and embarrassing herself. Twice during this hour-long session she had to excuse herself to go to the bathroom; her anxieties and fears had kindled a need to urinate.

While Michael held points on her lower back (B 23, B 47) and belly (CV 4, CV 5, CV 6), Meredith compared the experience of merging into traffic with trying to join into the rhythm of a jump rope. "I was never good at jump rope; I was unable to jump with the rhythm of the rope. Kids teased me all the time, and the pressure and ridicule made trusting my motor coordination difficult. I think my fear about merging into traffic is connected with the teasing I got about jump roping."

Michael encouraged Meredith to breathe slowly and deeply into her belly, as she visualized herself merging successfully into traffic. Re-creating this driving experience while receiving acupressure enabled her to gain a renewed sense of trust in herself.

Panic is what you feel when you get scared by your own emotions and don't have the skills to calm yourself down. Or when you're trying like mad to suppress feelings or memories.

— Ellen Bass & Laura Davis
The Courage to Heal

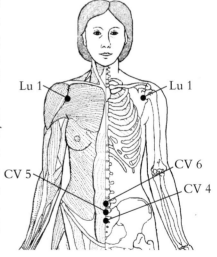

She was guided to visualize places along the highway to stop and use the restroom. Her anxiety about having to urinate became an empowering awareness to take care of herself. The deep relaxation from acupressure enabled her to communicate with her scared, anxious inner child, while the adult part of her was able to respond to the fears at the root of her anxiety.

Meredith learned self-acupressure and Kegel exercises (squeezing her rectum and buttock muscles multiple times) to strengthen her bladder. She also incorporated deep breathing exercises into her daily self-care routine. After several weeks, she no longer suffered from road anxiety; acupressure enabled her to trust and care for her inner child.

DIETARY CONSIDERATIONS

- **Enjoy Greens:** Green vegetables supply the body with a large quantity of B vitamins to calm anxiety.

- **Increase Grains:** Grains will give you an ample amount of B vitamins, which have a calming effect on the nervous system.

- **Foods to Avoid:** Sugar, salt, artificial colorings, white flour, additives, and preservatives can weaken your body. These debilitating foods, especially sugar, can make your anxiety and panic attacks worse. Food cooked with a moderate amount of salt is not harmful, but adding salt or soy sauce directly to your food at the table can create an internal imbalance.

QUICK TIPS FOR ANXIETY & PANIC ATTACKS

During an anxiety or panic attack, concentrate on breathing slowly and deeply while you hold the following acupressure points:

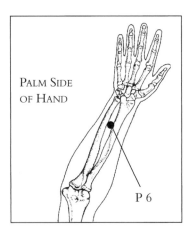

PALM SIDE
OF HAND

P 6

Inner Gate (P 6): Releasing the Inner Gate (in the middle of the inside of the forearm, three finger-widths above the wrist crease) relieves nausea, anxiety, racing heartbeat, and wrist pain. It is also known to balance the inner being.

Sea of Tranquility (CV 17): When an anxiety attack occurs, Sea of Tranquility (on the center of your breastbone), is the single best point to use for relief. Find the indentation in the breastbone, four finger-widths up from its base, to hold with your fingertips. As you gently press CV 17, concentrate on taking slow, deep breaths into your heart for three minutes. This emotional balancing point opens the chest for deep breathing, activates the thymus gland, and is especially good for counteracting anxiety, nervousness, panic, anguish, depression, hysteria, and other emotional imbalances.

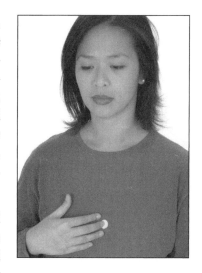

Letting Go (Lu 1): If you feel a panic attack coming on, use all of your fingertips to hold the upper, outer chest area on both sides, three finger-widths below the collarbone. Hold firmly, and concentrate on breathing deeply. Continue holding the Letting Go points for three minutes with the intention of moving through the panic period. Breathing deeply while holding these points can comfort and instantly calm an attack.

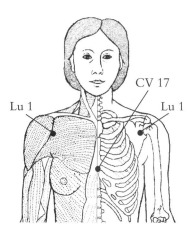

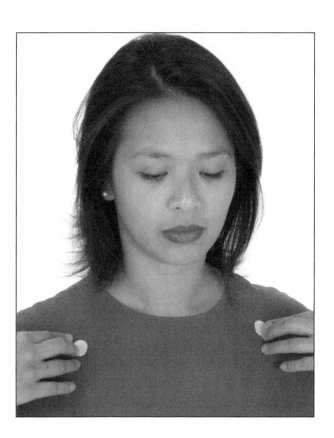

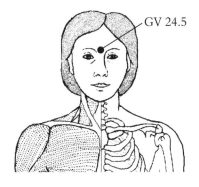

GV 24.5

Third Eye (GV 24.5): Another point for counteracting anxiety is located between the eyebrows, in the hollow spot where the bridge of the nose meets the ridge of the forehead. You can use this point most effectively by holding it lightly with your eyes closed, concentrating on the touch between your eyebrows. Holding the Third Eye in this way stimulates hormones and neurochemicals through the pituitary gland for relieving anxiety.

Try bringing the palms of your hands together in front of your chest. Then use your middle and index fingers to lightly touch the Third Eye point, between your eyebrows. Close your eyes, and take long, slow, deep breaths, concentrating on where you are touching for two minutes. Touching the Third Eye point calms the body and relieves nervousness, increasing intuition and emotional balance.

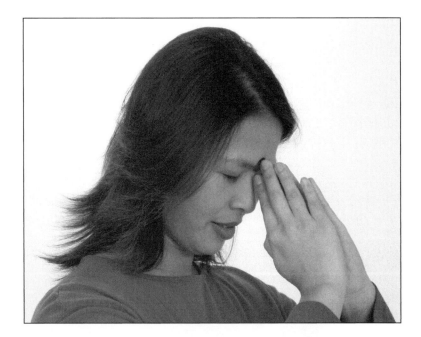

SELF-CARE ROUTINE FOR
ANXIETY & PANIC ATTACKS

As you practice the following self-care routine and deep breathing exercises, be aware of your thoughts and feelings. These acupressure points can give you new insights to help you overcome anxiety and panic attacks. Begin by lying down on your back comfortably.

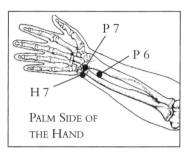

PALM SIDE OF
THE HAND

Step 1

Hold P 6 & P 7, Then Press H 7: P 6 and P 7 are located in the center, three and four finger-widths from the inner wrist crease, respectively. H 7 is on the inner wrist crease below the little finger. Hold each of these wrist points one at a time with your thumb for one minute. Breathe deeply into your belly to gain the benefits of these antianxiety points. Then switch sides.

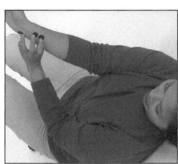

Step 2

Rock on the Middle Back: Place your feet flat on the floor, one shoulder-width apart. Interlace your fingers behind your head. Bring your head upward with your elbows pointing forward. Roll your upper body from side to side in this position for a minute. End by placing your hands on your lower abdominal area; breathe deeply, and relax for at least a minute.

Variation: With your head resting on the ground, raise your buttocks up into the air. As your buttocks come slowly downward, raise your head up using your arm muscles. Adjust this movement to press the muscles in your mid-back region. Continue alternating this up-and-down movement for one minute.

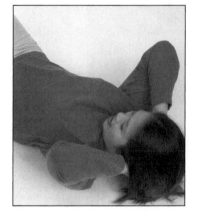

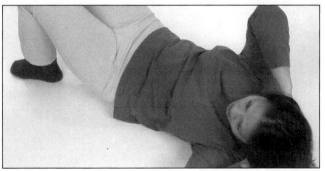

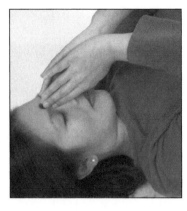

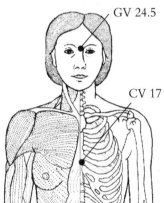

GV 24.5

CV 17

Step 3

Touch GV 24.5: Close your eyes, and bring your palms together. Use your middle and index fingers to lightly touch the Third Eye point (between your eyebrows in the hollow area where the bridge of the nose meets the ridge of your forehead). Close your eyes and take long, slow, deep breaths as you concentrate on this point for two minutes.

Step 4

Press Sea of Tranquility (CV 17): Keeping your palms together, press the backs of your thumbs against your breastbone, at the level of your heart. Keep your eyes closed, and concentrate on breathing slowly. Make each breath longer and deeper than the last one. After two minutes of deep breathing, let your hands drift down into your lap and sit quietly. Feel the vitality of your breath circulating through your entire body.

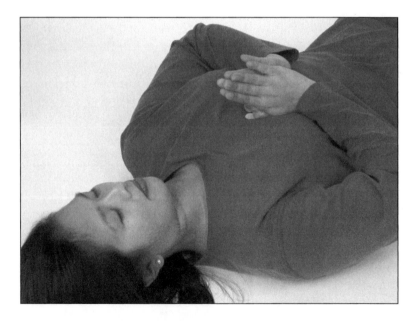

9

CODEPENDENCY

Codependency begins early in life. Most codependent individuals are survivors of dysfunctional relationships with their parents. Commonly alcohol, drugs, work, or sexual abuse consumed these parents. The children, whose basic emotional needs are not met during their developmental stages, grow up seeking validation of their self-worth, attempting to re-create the parent-child relationship with others. They may even twist reality by inventing fantasies in an attempt to be loved.

Poor self-image, shame, and guilt develop; low self-esteem undercuts their ability to trust. In the end these patterns undermine their feelings of self-worth or success. Codependent people can become negatively absorbed with the lives and problems of others. They seem to know how the "targets" of their love and attention feel at all times, in the process losing touch with their own feelings, personal boundaries, and needs.

For codependent personalities, living through someone else's problems and emotions seems to be the only validation of their life purpose, sense of being lovable, and self-identity. When negative attitudes and distrust become the foundation for adulthood, the pain and instability of abandonment reinforces failure in intimacy.

A codependent person can also become easily overwhelmed and manipulated by charismatic personalities, positions of power, and sexual relationships. Codependent people often create a dependent role with teachers, therapists, medical providers, and religious leaders. Since they are prone to power imbalance, professionals need to be sensitive to this issue and establish clear boundaries in their work. Infatuation distorts boundaries, confuses intentions, and can trigger past emotional wounds.

Codependency is tricky because it brings on feelings of responsibility and loss of control over one's own feelings and life, not to speak of anger, jealousy, resentment, and guilt over the

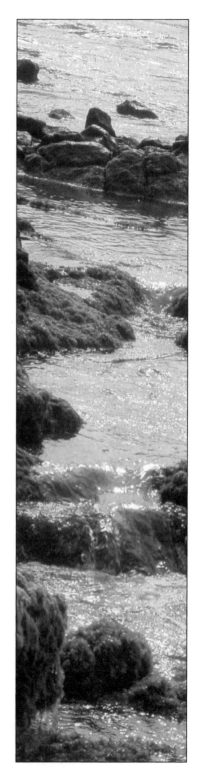

Affirmations to Counteract Codependency

- *I am lovable and deserve healthy relationships.*

- *I trust myself to make good choices.*

- *I am self-reliant and independent.*

- *I let go of trying to fix other people.*

- *I am open to the abundance and blessings of the universe.*

other person's issues. It is easier for them to identify with other people than with themselves, so not all codependent people who need help get it. But ever since the journalist (and codependent) Melody Beattie popularized codependence in her writings during the mid-1980s, millions of people have become better attuned to the symptoms and to the potential for healing.

Acupressure provides a codependent person with a safe, healthy way to explore and resolve emotional pain and buried feelings. Holding points releases muscle tension, increases circulation, and heightens a codependent person's self-awareness. Holding emotional balancing points for a longer period of time works through each layer of tension, bringing the body into balance. In Chapter 2 we saw how Judy, a woman in her forties with a thirty-year history of abusive relationships, used acupressure to heal emotional scars from her parents' bitter divorce. Lisa is another woman who used acupressure to heal her codependency pattern.

Lisa, a middle-aged wife, social worker, and mother of three, grew up in a dysfunctional, alcoholic home. Her mother was depressed and negative; her father was absent, out drinking and drunk most of the time. Lisa was the only girl in her family of four children. Although she did not draw her father's physical rage, he abused everyone else in the family on a daily basis.

Lisa found sanctuary in the other family members, by taking care of everything and everyone. She learned very young that if she did so, her father would leave her alone. Although this survival strategy saved her from physical harm, it did not fulfill her need for love and affection. Indeed, Lisa's mother and siblings withheld love from her because they were resentful that the father favored Lisa as the family caregiver.

Like many codependents, Lisa fell in love and married an alcoholic. She was eighteen. Two years later she was diagnosed with Crohn's disease, a chronic inflammation of the digestive tract that usually occurs in the small intestine and symptomatically affects every part of digestion. Crohn's disease has no cure, although drug treatments, surgery, nutritional supplements, and a mind-body approach can help individuals manage their symptoms.

Lisa had several surgeries over the years, as well as psychotherapy and medication for pain management and resulting symptoms of depression. Ten years later Lisa's flare-ups would still cause her so much discomfort that she could barely walk though the door to meet Beth Henning for her first acupressure session.

Acupressure helped Lisa become more comfortable physically and discharge emotionally painful memories from childhood. Muscle tension stored layers and layers of deep feelings. Holding CV 12 and CV 17, while breathing deeply, gave her the strength and courage to explore her trauma and stress. These points also helped release diaphragmatic tension and pain, two debilitating symptoms often reported clinically by Crohn's sufferers. Daily deep breathing practices also helped to free her feelings of betrayal.

Holding the emotional balancing points P 6, CV 17, and CV 6 helped Lisa to relax and reflect on her past, back to her earliest memories of childhood. These calming points transformed the feelings and images of her mother's and brothers' scorn and neglect and replaced them with an awareness of her own goodness. The Cross Hug exercise, described later in this chapter, supported her to safely relive a traumatic memory. After her acupressure sessions Lisa felt peaceful, relaxed, and fulfilled, with a new and healthy sense of purpose she had never experienced before.

With just a few weeks of regular practice three times per day, Lisa's stomach pains and indigestion calmed down and remained stable. She became symptom free after four months of daily self-care, to the surprise of her family, doctors, and therapists. She later went on to study acupressure and alternative modalities with Beth. She now thrives in her own holistic healing practice, applying touch therapies, shamanism, and the lessons of her own experiences to help others.

Healing codependency requires a multifaceted program integrating bodywork, psychotherapy, spiritual practice, and a support team of loving family and friends. Codependent behavior is an instinctive response to unhealthy, unpredictable, and emotionally unstable situations. Although these responses may seem dysfunctional and self-defeating at times, try not to be self-judgmental. Be patient and loving as you create new visions for your life.

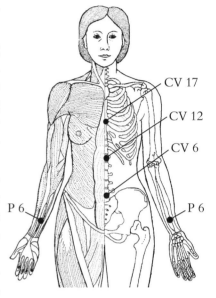

If you are willing to allow the energy of the universe to move through you by trusting and following your intuition you will increase your sense of aliveness and your body will reflect this with increasing health, beauty, and vitality.

— Shakti Gawain
Creative Visualization

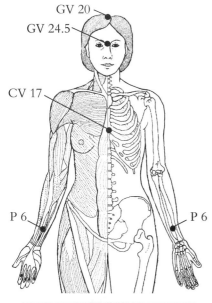

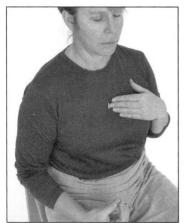

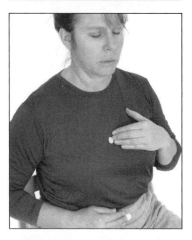

DIETARY CONSIDERATIONS

Clients with codependent patterns often use food to stuff feelings and avoid emotional pain. Dietary changes can be an important part of recovering from addictive patterns. Experiment with the following suggestions, and refer to Chapter 26 for further information.

- **Sugar:** Eliminate white sugar from your diet. Limit your fruit intake, especially tropical and citrus fruits. Increase healthy sweets like squash, baked yam, apples, and carrots.

- **Decrease Dairy Products:** Dairy products can be congesting. Since they can numb feelings and bloat the body, consider eating less when you are going through the process of deep emotional healing.

- **Yeast:** Yeast often causes allergic reactions. Toasting bread and other grains can help digest foods containing yeast.

- **Increase Greens:** Greens, rich in minerals and vitamins, increase vitality and boost your immune system. Be careful eating spinach, especially if osteoporosis is present, since this leafy green can inhibit calcium absorption.

QUICK TIPS FOR CODEPENDENCY

Cross Hug: Cross your hands at your heart, and hug yourself with deep breathing for two minutes.

Hold CV 17 with Thumb & Third Fingertips: Hold CV 17 with your left fingertips on the indentation in the center of your breastbone. With your right hand, touch your right thumb and third fingertip together. Hold these points with your eyes closed as you breathe deeply for two minutes.

Hold CV 17 with CV 6: Continue to hold CV 17 as your right hand presses CV 6 (located three finger-widths below the navel). As you breathe deeply, relax for two minutes.

Hold P 6: Hold this point (located three finger-widths above your wrist crease) to nurture your inner and outer awareness.

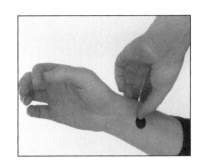

To transform codependency, vow to support your inner healing by practicing self-acupressure on a regular daily basis.

SELF-CARE ROUTINE FOR CODEPENDENCY

Using the following step-by-step guidelines, you can heal painful emotional wounds at your own pace in the privacy of your home. For safety, we suggest that you have a trustworthy friend or therapist present for emotional support and guidance. This self-care routine significantly reduces emotional stress.

Find a comfortable position on your back using pillows, blankets, soft lighting, and music to encourage deep relaxation. Hold each of the following points for two minutes.

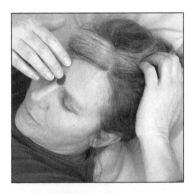

Step 1

Hold GV 20 with GV 24.5: Place your right hand on the top of your head to lightly touch GV 20. Place your left fingertips lightly on the Third Eye point (GV 24.5, between your eyebrows), and breathe deeply for two minutes. This clears your mind and increases your intuition.

Step 2

Hold GV 20 with CV 17: Continue holding GV 20 with the right hand while you place your left hand on the center of the breastbone for emotional and mental clarity. Breathe deeply as you hold these points for two minutes, paying attention to your feelings and images to generate self-love and spiritual healing.

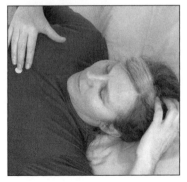

Step 3

Hold GV 20 with CV 12: Continue to hold GV 20 with your right hand, and move your left hand to the center of your belly. Apply slow, steady pressure to these points for two minutes. This point combination harmonizes your sense of self and heightens self-awareness and courage.

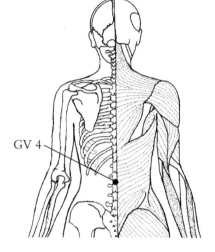

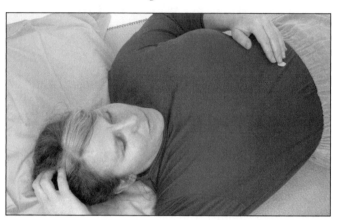

Step 4

Hold GV 20 with CV 6: Continue to hold GV 20 with your right hand, and move your left hand three finger-widths below the belly button. Apply slow, steady pressure and breathe deeply for two minutes to enhance your healing energy. Holding these points encourages the release of fear and tension related to abandonment and survival.

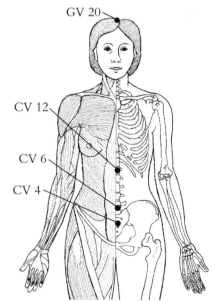

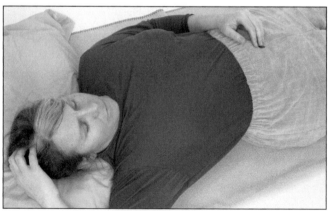

Step 5

Hold GV 20 with GV 4: Continue to hold GV 20 with your right hand, and move your left hand underneath your back at waist level for two minutes. If finger pressure is uncomfortable, slide your palm underneath your lower back area to open the point. The Gate of Life (GV 4) stores the inherited gifts of your ancestors and increases inner strength.

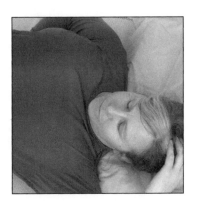

Step 6

Deeply Relax: Cover yourself with a blanket, and place your hands over your lower belly. Deeply relax for ten minutes. Breathe deeply to rejuvenate your body and rebalance your emotional well-being.

You do not have to hold all of these points to receive a benefit. Holding one or two can be effective.

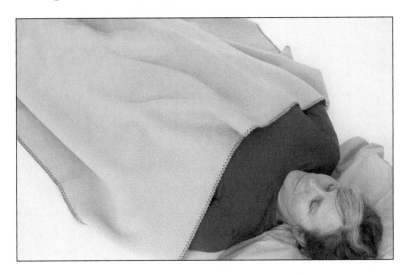

Whoever forces it spoils it.

Whoever grasps it loses it.

— Lao Tzu
The Art & Practice of Loving

10

DEPRESSION

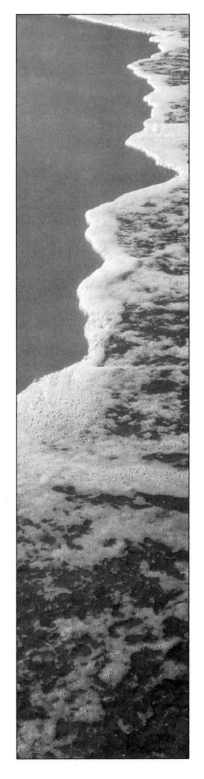

Depression is one of the most common health problems in all age groups. But, individuals with short-term, run-of-the-mill depression often do not recognize the disorder or know how to alleviate it, despite the enormous amount of media attention depression has received. For chronic depression, involving antidepressant drugs (see Preface), professional psychotherapy is necessary. We have found that a holistic approach using acupressure, diet, daily exercise, therapy, and self-awareness training increases the likelihood of integrating significant life changes successfully.

Depression signals that something in your life is out of balance and needs your attention. In depression, mood and interest drop dramatically from normal levels. One of the major symptoms is self-absorption, dwelling on sadness, emptiness, and how awful life feels. Depressed people usually have physical symptoms like poor concentration, decreased sex drive, changes in weight, appetite, and sleep patterns. Sluggish metabolism and shallow breathing often accompany depression. A negative view develops that may include hopelessness about the future, discouragement, and feelings of worthlessness. Depression is a despondent feeling, often carrying a badge of shame and guilt that exacerbates low morale and poor self-esteem.

Many factors can contribute to depression, including environmental and social stress, lack of purpose, unfulfilling relationships, poor or inadequate exercise, poor nutrition and eating habits, medical conditions, chronic pain, personality traits, changes in brain chemistry, and genes. Sometimes a hormone imbalance, such as an abnormality in the function of the thyroid or adrenal gland, can play a role in causing depression.

For those who have severe depression and are having trouble getting motivated to implement healthy lifestyle changes, taking

Affirmations to Counteract Depression

- *I am being taken care of.*

- *I let go of my expectations.*

- *I love myself for what I am going through.*

- *I open my heart to love and the joys of life.*

- *I am thankful for all I have.*

medications may help to clear the way to pursue acupressure. We have seen people on antidepressant medications benefit greatly from acupressure, so much so that they were able to gradually get off medications completely. Acupressure increases circulation and can expand the absorption of medications; thus, after receiving acupressure, patients on antidepressants often feel overmedicated. Be sure to consult with your doctor if you have any questions about your dosage. A smaller dosage prescribed by your doctor would mean that your body chemistry is rebalancing.

The antidepressant acupressure points release emotional distress, enabling you to relax and rebalance the neurochemistry of your body. As acupressure points are held and the person breathes slowly and deeply, the body relaxes and is able to let go of repressed emotions. Counseling and therapy can also help process the roots of depression and support positive life changes.

When Mark, an editor for a small publishing company on the West Coast, first sought help for his depression, he was living what could only be described as a dangerously unhealthy lifestyle. He spent long hours every day sitting at his computer, he rarely exercised, and he ate his biggest meal of the day late at night. He enjoyed fast foods high in fat, sugar, and salt. Insomnia, anxiety, and upper respiratory symptoms also afflicted him. His string of unsuccessful relationships with women made him feel and believe that he was unlovable.

Mark had been an active person earlier in his life, but his depression became so incapacitating that he sought out psychotherapy, choosing a cognitive therapist who specialized in depression. Once Mark understood how his poor habits and physical symptoms contributed to his depression, he began to engage himself in therapy wholeheartedly. Over the course of seven sessions he discovered how his family dynamics had contributed to his insecurities and dependencies. He began to recognize the recurring patterns in his unwise decisions, particularly with women, but also in other parts of his life. During this time he also learned new skills for cultivating intimate relationships. Mark started to break the cycle of depression; his outlook improved, and he began to care about himself.

Therapy, while valuable, didn't clear up all Mark's physical symptoms. Therefore his therapist referred him for acupressure, to work in conjunction with his ongoing psychotherapy. While receiving acupressure in a deep, relaxed state, Mark saw even more clearly that his old debilitating attitudes were connected to his childhood insecurities and fears. After processing these deep emotions in his acupressure sessions, he fell asleep. When he awoke, he felt remarkably relaxed and could breathe more deeply and freely than he had in a very long time. These experiences within his body renewed his self-esteem and transformed his feelings of inadequacy. His depression seemed to lift away. After four weekly acupressure sessions, his upper respiratory symptoms diminished as well as his insomnia and anxiety.

Mark practiced the self-care routines and discovered that they produced the same deep relaxation when combined with light stretching and aerobics. The more he moved his body and practiced deep breathing, the happier he felt. Mark also found new dietary principles instrumental in his healing process, covered in Chapter 26. After three months of intense weekly psychotherapy, Mark continued seeing his therapist and acupressure practitioner biweekly for maintenance and support, and to integrate his insights.

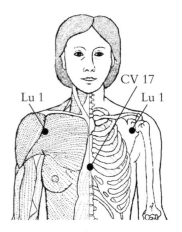

QUICK TIPS FOR DEPRESSION

Apply any of the following practices at any time. All you need is a few minutes; you don't have to practice all of them. Explore which ones give you the best results for counteracting your depression.

Hold Your Heart: Sit comfortably in a chair, or kneel on the floor. Place the heel of your hand on the center of your breastbone to hold the Sea of Tranquility (CV 17). Place your other hand over this hand to support your chest firmly. Tuck your head as you bend and relax your upper body down and forward. Begin long, slow, deep breathing with your eyes closed for two minutes.

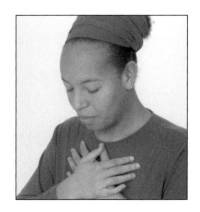

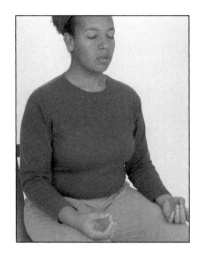

Deep Breathing Meditation: Depression can result from an inadequate supply of oxygen in the blood. Deep breathing and acupressure increase blood circulation and oxygen supply. Practice the following breathing meditation in a quiet spot, either indoors or out in nature. Sit comfortably with your spine straight. Touch your thumb and middle fingers together. Close your eyes and begin long, slow, deep breathing. As you focus your attention on your breath, prolong the inhalation with the intention to receive healing energy. Imagine that each slow exhalation releases burdens and past hurts. Focus on how each deep breath strengthens your ability to take care of yourself. Continue this breathing meditation for five to ten minutes.

Finger Position: This exercise activates potent points to better assimilate oxygen into your system. Hold your right thumb firmly with your left hand for two minutes. Then squeeze your right little finger firmly as you continue to breathe slowly and deeply for an additional two minutes. Switch sides to hold your left thumb and then your left little finger for two minutes each. Holding these fingers opens the breath and facilitates your ability to let go and receive healing energy.

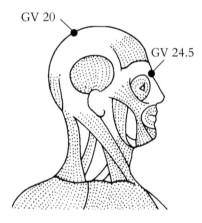

GV 20

GV 24.5

Hot & Cold Shower: After a hot shower, decrease the water temperature as low as you can tolerate. Cold water stimulates the nerves close to the surface of the skin and is rejuvenating. (However, women who are menstruating or pregnant should keep themselves warm.)

Acupressure Journal: Take five minutes and write down everything you're feeling. Express yourself. Write down a stream of thoughts without judgments. After five to ten minutes of journal writing, tear up or burn the pages to finalize the letting go of your feelings, or else save your writing to refer to later on. Try both ways to find out which style suits you best.

ACUPRESSURE
EMOTIONAL BALANCING STEPS

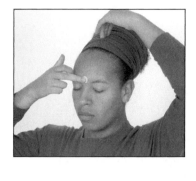

1. **Hold GV 20 with GV 24.5:** Place your right hand on the Hundred Meeting point (GV 20, on the top of your head), and your left hand at the Third Eye point (GV 24.5). Close your eyes, and breathe deeply for two minutes.

2. **Touch GV 20 with CV 17:** Move your left hand to the Sea of Tranquility (CV 17, located at the center of the breast-bone). Continue to breathe deeply for an additional minute.

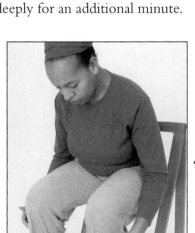

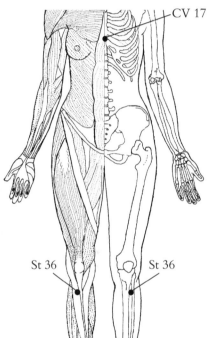

3. **Rub Both St 36:** Briskly rub the Three Mile point (St 36) on both legs. This rejuvenating point is located on the out-side of the shinbone, four finger-widths below the kneecap. Then hold the Three Mile point firmly for one minute.

4. **Stretch & Shake:** Stand up, stretch your body, and shake it out.

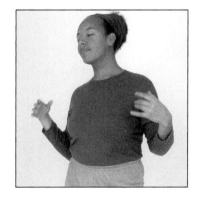

SELF-CARE ROUTINE FOR DEPRESSION
(STANDING)

The following routine stimulates acupressure points by stretching and expanding the chest to increase the assimilation of oxygen. This activates energy flow through meridians, the channels of energy that connect the acupressure points. As we mentioned earlier, when your meridians are blocked, you can become fatigued and despondent because your supply of energy is impaired. These exercises will energize your respiratory system, increase your lung capacity, and free tight shoulder muscles. Practice them in a comfortable standing position.

Step 1

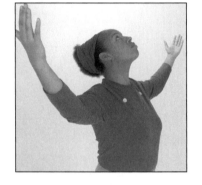

Opening Up & Letting Go: Use your fingertips to press the Letting Go point (Lu 1, on both sides of the upper, outer portion of your chest, three finger-widths below the collarbone). Inhale deeply as you gradually release your finger pressure, bring your arms outward, lift your chest, and tilt your head back. Hold your breath for a few seconds to assimilate the oxygen. Exhale as your head comes downward and your fingers return to Lu 1. Repeat this exercise five more times. Holding the Letting Go point counteracts depression by increasing your body's ability to breathe more deeply and assimilate oxygen.

Step 2

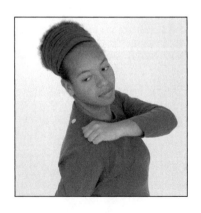

Swinging Fists from Shoulders to Buttocks:★ Stand comfortably with your feet a shoulder-width apart and your knees slightly bent. Twist your hips from side to side, allowing both arms to swing freely. Completely relax your arms and upper body as you swing. As you turn to the right, bend your left arm to gently tap your right shoulder, the Shoulder Well point (GB 21). Swing your right fist around your back to pound your left buttock, the Womb and Vitals point (B 48), simultaneously. As

---

★This exercise is beneficial if you do not have severe lower back pain or lower disk problems. If you do, do not twist your body. Instead, use your fist to pound your shoulders and your buttock muscles without twisting.

your upper body twists to your left, swing your right fist up onto your left shoulder (GB 21), as your left fist swings behind you to tap your right buttock (B 48). Continue to swing from side to side, alternating your fists to pound your shoulders and the opposite buttocks for one minute. This twisting exercise stimulates elimination. Without proper elimination, your system gets sluggish, unresponsive, and depressed.

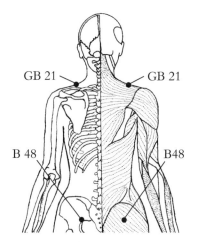

Step 3

Upper Back Opener:★ Continue standing comfortably with your feet a shoulder-width apart and knees slightly bent. Bring your hands behind the base of your spine, and interlace your fingers with your palms facing each other. Gradually bend forward, bringing your upper body down with your legs straight. Inhale deeply as you raise your arms, flexing your chest out. Breathe deeply for at least a half-minute. This stretches the upper back and stimulates the emotional balancing acupressure points (B 36–B 38) between your shoulder blades, which are associated with depression as well as insomnia. Let your arms relax downward as they swing by your sides with your knees bent. Bend your knees and slowly come up using your thigh muscles to return to a standing position.

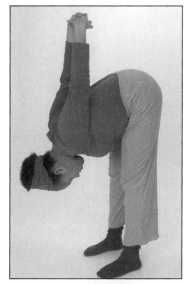

Step 4

Pounding Buttocks & Backs of Legs: Make fists to pound your buttocks. Bend your knees, and pound down the backs of your legs. With your knees bent, slowly pound up the back of your legs to your buttocks as you gradually come upward into a standing position. Continue for one minute. This stimulates a series of Bladder meridian points (B 48–B 54) for counteracting depression.

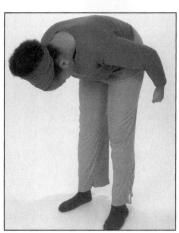

★If you have high blood pressure or cardio-vascular problems, see your doctor before doing this exercise.

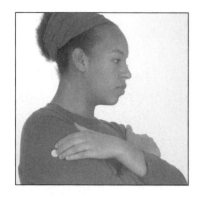

Step 5

Hug Twist:★ Hug yourself by reaching your arms around the front of your body. Grasp hold of the Upper Arm points (LI 14) on the sides of your upper arms one-third of the way down from the tip of your shoulders to your elbows. With your feet a shoulder-width apart, twist your upper body from one side to the other as you breathe deeply for half a minute.

Step 6

Opening Up & Letting Go: Come full cycle by repeating the breathing exercise described in Step 1 for two minutes.

SELF–CARE ROUTINE FOR DEPRESSION
(LYING DOWN)

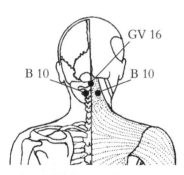

WINDOWS OF THE SKY POINTS

The following routine uses self-massage, movement, deep breathing, and acupressure to counteract depression. This combination stimulates the release of endorphins, the body's natural painkillers that produce euphoric, uplifting feelings and can alleviate depression. The last few steps use emotional balancing points in a breathing movement meditation that can change a depressed metabolism, leaving you feeling calm and peaceful.

Find a private place to practice without distractions. Dim the lights. Make sure the room is warm and draft free. Lie down on your back with your knees bent, feet flat on the floor, comfortably apart.

GV 16
B 10   B 10

Step 1

Neck Massage: Knead the muscles of your neck firmly. Curve your fingers, placing your fingertips on both sides of your upper neck (B 10). Use the heel of your hand to press the outside of your neck and gradually squeeze the neck muscles. Keep your eyes closed, and concentrate on breathing deeply while you massage your neck and shoulders for two minutes. This neck massage stimulates the Windows of the Sky points, which are traditionally used to relieve depression. These points open the energy flow through the neck, forming a bridge that links the mind and body.

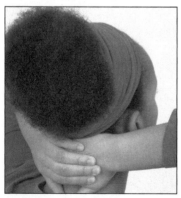

★Do not twist your body if you have lower back pain or a disk problem.

Step 2

Neck Press & Stretch: Interlace your fingers securely over your neck. Inhale as you lift your chest, bring your elbows upward, and move your head back slowly. Exhale as your head relaxes down and your elbows come close together. Use the heels of your hands to press and release chronic neck tension. Breathe slowly and deeply, inhaling up and exhaling down for two minutes. Then lower your head gently, and bring your hands to your belly. Keeping your eyes closed; roll your head slowly from side to side. This exercise further releases the antidepression Windows of the Sky points. Deep breathing in this posture also benefits the thyroid gland and balances the metabolism.

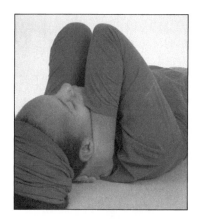

Step 3

Skull Press: Place the heels of your hands on the sides of your head. Bring your elbows outward and apply pressure slowly into the center of your skull. Apply direct, firm pressure on various areas of the skull at five-second intervals for a total of one minute. Then use your fingertips and nails to vigorously rub all areas of your skull. This exercise releases the Gall Bladder meridian, associated with depression, headaches, indecision, and judgmental attitudes.

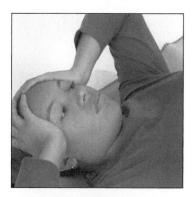

Step 4

Touch GB 14: Lightly place your middle fingers on your forehead to gently hold the emotional balancing GB 14 point. (This point is located one finger-width above the center of the eyebrow, in line with the iris of the eye.) Breathe deeply as you touch GB 14 for one minute, clearing emotional distress and enhancing morale.

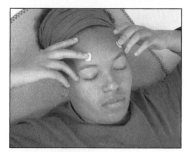

Step 5

Hold CV 17: Place the heel of one hand against the center of your breastbone at the level of your heart, to press the Sea of Tranquility point (CV 17). Place your other hand over that hand for support, and breathe deeply for one minute. Holding this point harmonizes the emotions and relieves anxiety, depression, confusion, and nervousness.

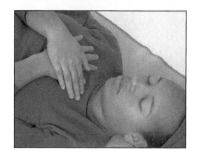

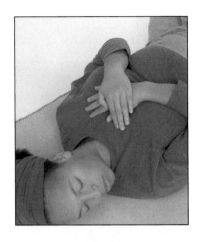

Step 6

Hands on Heart Twist: Remain lying on your back with your knees bent, and keep your feet flat on the floor. With both hands over the center of your chest, slowly turn your head to the right as your knees fall to the left. Inhale deeply as your knees come back to center. Exhale as your head rolls to the left while your knees relax down to your right. Continue for one minute. This exercise opens the Gall Bladder meridian for dealing with judgments, indecision, headaches, and depression.

Roll onto your side and slowly pick yourself up into a comfortable sitting position for the next exercise.

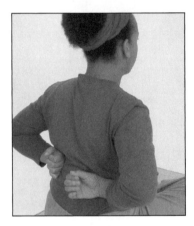

Step 7

Lower Back Rub: Place the backs of your hands against your lower back on both sides of your spine. Briskly rub up and down from your middle back down to your buttocks, to create heat from the friction, for one minute. This movement fortifies the kidneys and relieves exhaustion, fatigue, depression, paranoia, and fear.

Come to a comfortable standing position with your hands crossed over your chest.

Step 8

Opening Up & Letting Go: Place your fingertips on the upper, outer sides of your chest, three finger-widths below your outer collarbone, to press the Letting Go points (Lu 1). Inhale deeply as your hands come out to the sides and your head tilts back. Inhale more as you stretch back for a few seconds. Exhale, returning to Lu 1. Continue for two minutes to reduce depression, expand your lung capacity, and restore your well-being.

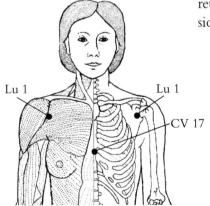

Lu 1   Lu 1

CV 17

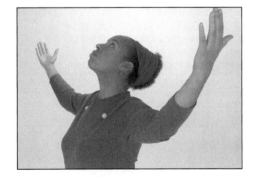

PREVENTING DEPRESSION

Each of the essential lifestyle factors listed here can affect depression. Reflect on how you can cultivate these aspects in your own life.

Work & Personal Growth: Meaningless work that lacks purpose can cause depression. If you have a job that makes you depressed, explore what type of work you would find more satisfying. A vocational counselor can help you explore various alternative types of work, suggest training resources, and open new opportunities.

Aerobic Exercise: Twenty minutes of jogging, swimming, brisk walking, or bicycling each day can prevent and relieve minor depression. Vigorous aerobic exercise necessitates deep breathing and thus counteracts depression.

Environmental Considerations: Gloomy surroundings can perpetuate depression. Some people need to live or work in an environment that has abundant natural light and fresh air. Improvements like installing a mirror to reflect more light or a fan for ventilation can contribute to good health.

Healthy Relationships: Friendships fulfill many human needs. If you tend to get depressed, seek opportunities to meet positive people who are likely to share your interests.

Future Plans & Goals: Planning to do something exciting in the future that you can look forward to can prevent depression.

Depression is a condition of energy depletion... It is possible to lose perspective and project depression onto unrelated areas of life, thinking that you are depressed because of this or that condition, instead of understanding the real cause: energy depletion... If you can accept and open to depression, you will recharge your energy reserves instead of suppressing the depression with self-rejection, such as becoming depressed about the depression.

— John Ruskan
Emotional Clearing

11

EMOTIONAL NUMBNESS

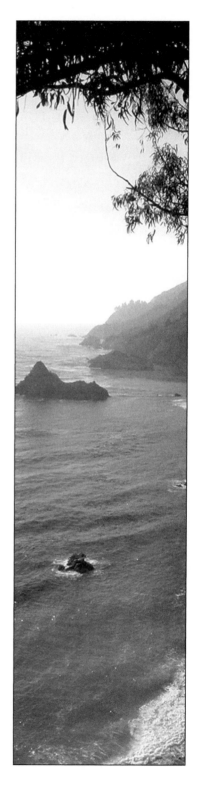

Numbness can be an adaptive response to a painful, threatening experience. The body is a complex organism capable of tremendous feeling and sensitivity. But the pain and shock of a traumatic experience can be so overwhelming to the senses that the body numbs itself for protection. The psyche can't handle the intensity of the trauma and thus shuts down emotionally in the moment, to process the event later. Emotional numbness and blocked feelings often continue long after the original traumatic event has ended; for instance, physical abuse from a parent can have residual effects long after childhood.

Pain causes muscles to contract, which inhibits circulation, prevents cells from receiving adequate nourishment, and limits the body's ability to access feeling. Pain, caused by an injury, disease, or functional disorder, is transmitted through the central nervous system, which activates neurochemical painkillers called endorphins. This biological safeguard from the shock of potentially dangerous situations can cause a person to *dissociate,* a word that psychologists and trauma specialists use to refer to what happens when a person becomes emotionally and/or physically numb. People who dissociate describe a feeling of "being out of their body" and detached from their environment, going through the motions of living with very little or no feeling.

Some people simply avoid their pain; for others, unresolved experiences or issues may trigger old emotional wounds that never healed. For example, if your parents argued with each other and were angry or screamed at you frequently when you were a child, you may have become particularly sensitive to raised voices. To protect yourself from the emotional pain of

Affirmations to Counteract Emotional Numbness

- *I am grateful to be alive.*

- *It is safe and healing for me to feel.*

- *I love my body and appreciate feeling.*

- *My vibrancy increases with each deep breath.*

- *I have tremendous feeling and sensitivity within me.*

being afraid and scared as a child, you may have unconsciously protected yourself by "tuning out" or "shutting down" whenever somebody shouts.

Avoiding people and places that are reminders of a trauma can cause emotional detachment and unresponsiveness. Detachment further disables the ability to resolve problems and emotional issues. Thus, the inability to feel becomes an obstacle to living a full and enriching life.

Processing the roots of trauma through psychotherapy and acupressure can transform emotional numbness; understanding the causes can be the first step. In addition, acupressure's healing touch cultivates greater body awareness and emotional sensitivity. When acupressure points are held, the tension dissolves and life energy flows through the body. Acupressure, along with guided visualization of the issues associated with numbness, can enable a person to reexperience and release the source of their trauma and become free to enjoy life more. Practicing relaxation methods are a big part of retraining the mind and body, which is why acupressure and deep breathing are so effective.

John, a successful businessman, inherited his parents' business after they died. His grief over their deaths, and the demands he faced with the growing business, led to a number of personal problems, which caused him tremendous stress. With mounting anxiety in his life, the frequency of his tension headaches increased until they were recurring almost every day. John's wife, Margaret, was seriously considering a divorce because he was not meeting her needs for emotional intimacy. John was unable to express his feelings or to show affection for his wife or anything else that mattered. The roots of his inability to express his inner feelings lay with his parents, who were not affectionate either. As a little boy, he learned to cut himself off from the pain and hurt of feeling unloved.

Margaret had good results with acupressure on two separate occasions: for relieving tennis elbow, and for recovery from bouts of depression. She encouraged John to try acupressure as a way of getting in touch with his feelings. At first, although he had seen his wife's success with acupressure, he was skeptical about its working for his problems; but he was motivated because he loved Margaret and wanted to save their relationship.

John was surprised by how much he enjoyed the deep relaxation he experienced from his sessions. When the points on his shoulders (GB 21) were being pressed, he described his tension as being like "rusty nails holding him back." He had to release this tension before he could relive and vanquish the sadness, shame, and hurt that had resulted from his father's ridicule thirty years earlier.

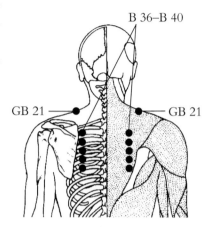

After just eight acupressure sessions, John was surprised at the remarkable difference he felt. He was able to cry for the first time in many years. In addition to his weekly sessions, John worked on himself at home, using tennis balls to press acupressure points between the shoulder blades (B 36–B 40). He also used points on his shoulders to help cope with work-related stress. His headaches faded and he was more at ease. Margaret credited his new vitality, better health, and their saved marriage to acupressure.

LIFESTYLE CAUSES OF NUMBNESS

Numbness isn't always a result of early childhood or adult trauma. Lifestyle factors can also play a major role in the numbing process.

Stress & Pace of Life: Emotional numbness commonly occurs from the overwhelming stresses of a busy life. Multiple distractions, not paying attention to your body, being in your head, and ignoring feelings can all result in numbness. A stressful environment constricts your muscles, shuts off circulation, and further depletes your energy.

Inadequate Exercise: The body gets lethargic and numb without use; exercise increases circulation and restores vitality.

Diet & Eating Habits: Excessively rich foods containing butter or cream and fried foods can cause congestion, slow down the metabolism, and dull your senses. Eating under stress can stuff your feelings. This further inhibits digestion as well as the absorption of nutrients and thus impairs vitality.

Environmental Conditions: Living in damp, dark, cloudy regions can be depressing. Chemical toxins and air pollution can cause shallow breathing, which in turn inhibits your body from feeling. Thus, repressive surroundings can dull your senses.

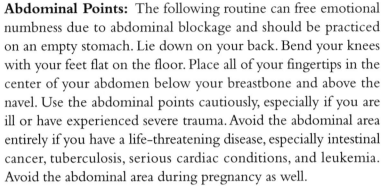

SUGGESTIONS FOR CULTIVATING EMOTIONAL SENSITIVITY

Abdominal Points: The following routine can free emotional numbness due to abdominal blockage and should be practiced on an empty stomach. Lie down on your back. Bend your knees with your feet flat on the floor. Place all of your fingertips in the center of your abdomen below your breastbone and above the navel. Use the abdominal points cautiously, especially if you are ill or have experienced severe trauma. Avoid the abdominal area entirely if you have a life-threatening disease, especially intestinal cancer, tuberculosis, serious cardiac conditions, and leukemia. Avoid the abdominal area during pregnancy as well.

Gradually apply moderate to firm pressure to your abdomen with all of your fingertips. Press in slowly and hold each position (CV 4–CV 14) for five seconds each, moving downward through the midline of the abdomen toward the public bone. Hold painful areas more gently as you focus on breathing slowly and deeply.★ Continue for two minutes. Be sure to deeply relax on your back with your eyes closed for five minutes immediately after using these abdominal points. In three months of daily practice, you may be surprised how much more alive you feel.

Dietary Considerations: Diet plays an important role in counteracting numbness. Processed, devitalized foods containing white flour, sugar, preservatives, and hydrogenated oils and fats all contribute to numbness. Eat more fresh vegetables and sprouts, particularly a variety of leafy greens. Eliminating coffee and red meat will increase your emotional sensitivity. Also, reduce your intake of dairy products, fried foods, and salt. Please refer to Chapter 26 for further information.

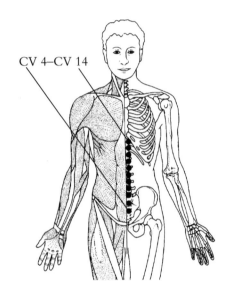

CV 4–CV 14

★Many emotionally numb women also have cysts that feel sore and tight. Do not hold these areas with any sort of deep pressure.

Movement: When trauma registers in your body, pain and stiffness can restrict your movements and lead to emotional numbness. These body dynamics affect your gestures, tone of voice, and facial expressions. To free up buried feelings, gently exaggerate whatever movements you are making. By taking a few minutes to effortlessly exaggerate your normal gestures and unconscious movements, you can gain new awareness to shift old patterns within yourself.

Stretching: Stretch your whole body several times a day. Yoga classes are excellent. After several months of daily stretching, you may notice a remarkable difference in how in tune you are with your body.

Aerobic Exercise: Daily aerobic exercise for twenty or thirty minutes—swimming, bicycling, running, or brisk walking—develops muscle tone, stimulates deep breathing, opens the pores of your skin, and increases blood circulation.

Deep Belly Breathing: Place one hand on your chest and the other on your lower belly. Close your eyes and focus your attention on your body. As you breathe deeply, imagine your breath nurturing your inner being to be more in touch with your feelings. Stay focused on the contact of your hands to regain more feeling in your body. Continue to breathe slowly and deeply in this way for three minutes.

It is always important for us to be aware of feelings. Our feelings exist for good reason and so deserve our attention and respect.

Even uncomfortable feelings that we might prefer to avoid, such as anger and depression, may serve to preserve the dignity and integrity of the self.

— Harriet Goldhor Lerner
The Dance of Intimacy

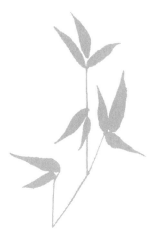

SELF-CARE ROUTINE FOR EMOTIONAL NUMBNESS

Two tennis balls are needed for the following self-care routine. Practice once or twice a day for a few weeks to regain awareness of your emotions.

Step 1

Lying on Tennis Balls: Place two tennis balls a couple of inches apart on a thick towel. Put a folded sock between the balls to separate them, and roll the balls up in a towel like a tight burrito. As an alternative to the towel, you can put the balls together in another sock.

Lie down on your back; bend your knees with your feet flat on the floor. Gently place the tennis balls underneath your upper back, centering them between your shoulder blades and the spine. If the pressure from the balls feels sharp or hurts, use a larger, thicker towel. If, on the other hand, you do not feel much of anything, then use a smaller, thinner towel or no towel at all. Close your eyes, and focus your attention on your chest or belly. As you breathe deeply into your heart, imagine your breath reawakening your feelings. Observe the sensations inside your body. Continue to breathe deeply for two minutes as you explore any sensations you may be feeling.

The disconnection between body and soul is one of the most important effects of trauma. Loss of skin sensation is a common physical manifestation of the numbness and disconnection people experience after trauma.

— Peter A. Levine
Waking the Tiger

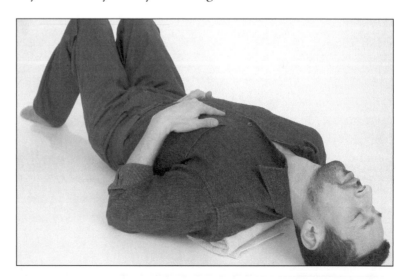

Step 2

Press Your Abdomen and Roll on Your Back: With your knees bent and your eyes closed, practice long, deep breathing, as you very slowly roll up and down over the balls for two minutes. This presses B 36, B 37, and B 38 for awakening emotional sensitivity. Gradually apply moderate to firm pressure with your fingertips on the center of your abdomen. Press in slowly, and hold CV 12 (midway between your navel and the base of your ribcage). Keeping your eyes closed, continue for a couple of minutes as you also focus your attention on the pressure in your upper back from the balls between your shoulder blades.

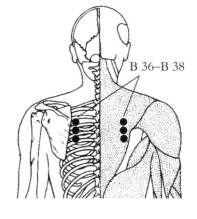

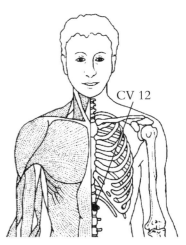

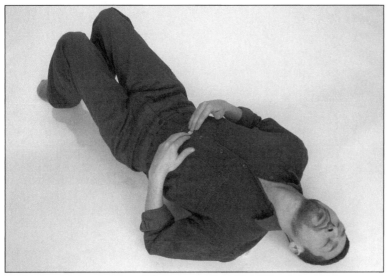

Step 3

Deep Relaxation: Immediately after you remove the tennis balls, cover yourself with a sheet or blanket and relax for five to ten minutes. Afterward spend a few minutes exploring your body awareness and noticing any sensations inside your chest and belly. Fostering greater sensitivity to your body comes from opening your acupressure points, breathing deeply, and spending time focusing on your body's awareness.

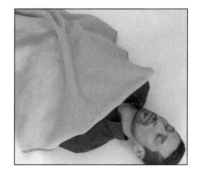

12

FEAR & PHOBIAS

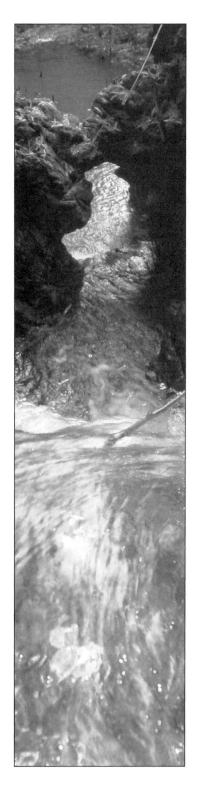

There are many types and degrees of fear. Our focus in this chapter is on phobias and common fears such as fear of failure, rejection, or abandonment, fear of not being loved, fear of not being heard, and fear of losing a loved one. Regularly practicing the exercises in this chapter will also prepare you to deal with fears related to severe trauma and violence. Fear triggers your deepest instincts to know your limits for handling dangerous and challenging situations.

When people are afraid, they often try to numb or medicate themselves by drinking alcohol, taking drugs, or overeating. The supportive touch of acupressure can help you become confident and courageous to face, rather than avoid, your fears. Public speaking, for instance, can be scary. Before you speak in front of people, take a few minutes to hold the Elegant Mansion points (K 27) on both sides directly below the top of your collarbone; this will enable you to clear your throat and breathe deeply to calm your fear. Use your thumb on one side, and your fingertips on the other side of the breastbone, in between the first and second ribs. Hold these chest points firmly, and breathe slowly and deeply when fear or anxiety surfaces in your work or in an intimate relationship. This practice can transform anxiety or a panic attack into an empowering, enriching experience. When you pay attention to your fear while breathing deeply, you become more creative and go deeper into expressing your inner being.

Fear is a natural response to danger, to a threat, or to an attack. Your body reacts to fear by contracting your muscles and respiratory system and restricting your breathing, causing anxiety. When you are scared, your heartbeat races and adrenaline increases. Without using the energy rush from adrenaline, the body freezes and becomes immobilized. The neck muscles contract and close the throat area. The lungs constrict, breathing gets shallow, and the voice loses the power of speech. When you stop breathing,

Affirmations to Counteract Fear & Phobias

- *I trust what I know is right.*

- *I am blessed and being taken care of.*

- *There is nothing to fear; all is well.*

- *I am grateful for what I have and who I am.*

- *I have the faith and courage to face whatever life presents.*

the cells of your body do not get nourished. Your inner awareness, sensory perceptions, and intuition decrease. Fear of the unknown contracts the musculature of your body and blocks your sensory awareness. Oxygen flow is essential for exploring deep feelings. So when fear arises, make a conscious choice to breathe deeply.

Courage to face the unknown cannot occur without deep breathing; your breath is a vehicle for empowerment. Conscious deep breathing can transform emotions and enable you to accept fear during your emotional healing process. Paying attention to the fullness of your breath can help you identify your emotional response.

Pressing the Sea of Tranquility (CV 17, on the center of your breastbone), can open your chest, facilitate breathing, and stabilize a panic or anxiety attack. This calming point is located four finger-widths above the base of the breastbone, in an indentation at the level of the heart. Let yourself relax and breathe through your nose if possible. Breathing slowly through your nose serves as a safety valve to prevent hyperventilation.

Your body registers multiple reactions during a traumatic experience. Over time emotional issues and memories may fade into the unconscious, but they don't disappear; they can become blocked and stored in the musculature, particularly in the back, buttocks, and shoulders. Back tension and stress are commonly related to fear. The back is difficult to reach, just as unconscious fear is difficult to recognize. Thus, releasing the acupressure points on the meridians that travel through the back can rebalance traumas, fears, and phobias.

Phobias

A phobia is a specific, persistent, irrational fear that can control your life, limit your actions, and stifle personal growth. There are many phobias, including fear of crowds, intimacy, heights, animals, bugs, isolation, water, confined spaces, being touched, darkness, and death, to name a few. Most phobic problems interfere with social, emotional, or occupational functioning and require treatment from a skilled psychotherapist, usually using behavior modification. Recurring phobias can be physically destructive and detrimental to your health. Phobias undermine self-confidence and sabotage self-expression, causing behavioral limitations.

Over time obsessive fears can develop into phobias, which can tax your body, causing chronic fatigue, panic attacks, and nightmares. Unresolved fear from traumatic past events can also become phobias. Extreme fear, terror, and pain can cause the mind to dissociate from reality, which throws the nervous system into conflict and can create phobias and, in severe cases, mental illness.

In traditional Chinese medicine, fear is associated with the kidneys. The kidneys not only filter water but also store the body's energy reserves. Fear stimulates adrenaline and the fight-or-flight response to a threatening situation. The adrenal glands are located directly above the kidneys. Adrenaline activates the body's energy reserves by stimulating the kidneys. A person who has persistent fears due to a phobia commonly suffers from chronic fatigue symptoms, back pain (where the kidneys are located), or nightmares. Thus, in traditional Chinese medicine, the strength of the kidneys governs your response to fear, whether it debilitates you or gives you courage to face your challenges. Strengthening the kidneys by using acupressure can similarly balance fear and phobias.

Acupressure's healing process can change a person's internal body chemistry by rebalancing the energy surging through the points and meridians. As you try to heal yourself in a safe environment, holding the points, your body deeply relaxes, enabling the breath and healing energy to open. This increases circulation; when blood flows optimally and nourishes body cells, your awareness becomes heightened. Over several months of applying acupressure, renewed body awareness and self-trust can be obtained. With the support of a psychotherapist to process past traumatic fears and phobias, an individual can heal past emotional wounds.

Just as your body is made by cells, your dreams are made by emotions. There are two main sources of those emotions. One is fear, and all the emotions that come from fear; the other is love, and all the emotions that come from love. We experience both emotions but the one that predominates in everyday people is fear.

— Don Miguel Ruiz
The Mastery of Love

Fear & Dyslexia

We believe that fear is one of the major causes of the learning disability known as dyslexia. Often dyslexia originates from a traumatic experience in a child's learning process. Children can be traumatized in school in a variety of ways. Calling on a child abruptly to perform in front of the class, mocking or ridiculing her appearance or behavior, can be devastating and weaken her self-confidence. These scary, hurtful events affect not only a child's emotions but also her physical well-being. For instance, fear can contract a child's shoulders and chest muscles, causing shallow breathing. His eyes can become fixated and lock up, affecting the optic nerve and his ability to distinguish the order of numbers or letters when reading. Certainly many other causes and symptoms are involved in dyslexia, too numerous to include here.

Love is letting go of fear.

— Gerald Jampolsky, MD
The Art and Practice of Loving

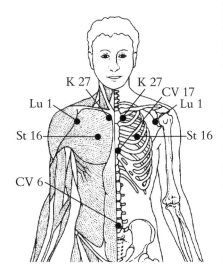

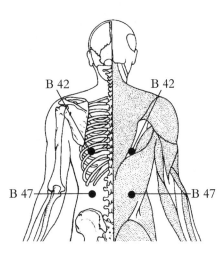

Gary, a successful middle-aged single businessman, had suffered from constant shoulder, neck, and back tension ever since the sudden death of his mother over a year before. Body pain forced him to turn down several lucrative conference and workshop opportunities. When physical therapy, psychotherapy, and spiritual counseling did not relieve his pain, he became fearful, which affected his livelihood.

Gary decided to explore acupressure as an alternative health option. His first session focused on upper body tension. He learned how to use deep breathing to relieve his stress and pain. Feelings about a past trauma surfaced during work on Lu 1, K 27, and St 16 in his upper chest area. Gary's memory took him back into his childhood, when he was preparing a speech in the third grade. He remembered his mother and sister mocking him for struggling so hard with the assignment. At this vulnerable age, Gary was attached to his mother for support, and the experience was traumatic for him. As he told the story, Gary's stomach and mid-back knotted up.

Holding the mid- and low back points B 42 and B 47, with CV 6 in the lower belly, revealed Gary's childhood fear about performance. For years he felt competitive with his younger sister, who was naturally adept at school and studying. When his sixth-grade teacher required him to take a battery of tests to determine whether he had a learning disorder, his mother began treating him with special care. Even through his college years, Gary and his mother were emotionally inseparable. Their relationship contributed to a pattern of overreliance on others in order to feel confident and safe. As a result, Gary's love relationships throughout his adult life suffered. No one ever measured up to his mother's coaching, love, and support.

An acupressure session or a specific event, such as Gary's mother's death, can trigger the release of deep, hidden emotions. Often the pain and tension we feel in our bodies is a cover for something deeper that is going on. Holding emotional balancing point CV 17 on the breastbone brought up Gary's deep feelings of grief at the loss of his mother, which also triggered his latent fear of not being able to perform. The stress of her death, along with his fear and lack of self-confidence, caused his body to contract and shake, releasing a range of emotions. His fear of facing the world without his mother caused Gary to cry softly before falling into a deep sleep.

Gary received three additional emotional balancing acupressure sessions and learned a self-acupressure routine. He practiced daily and wrote down his feelings in his journal for ten minutes each day. Within a month he was able to reasonably manage his emotions, handle his body pain, and resume his normal professional activities.

When the fear arises, which it does over and over again, it becomes a signal that it is time to let go, rebalance and find an unconditional allowing of life.

— Richard Moss, MD
The I That Is We

QUICK TIPS FOR FEAR & PHOBIAS

Hold Your Lower Back Points (B 23, B 47): Place your hands at your waist, with your thumbs on the ropelike muscles near the spine and your fingers wrapped around your sides. With your thumbs, apply firm, steady pressure in toward the spine on the outer edges of those ropy muscles, so that your thumbs are about four inches apart. This inward pressure stimulates B 47. You can also stimulate the inner point, B 23, by pressing the top of the large vertical muscles two finger-widths away from the spine. Use either your thumbs or your fingertips to stimulate one side at a time or both sides at once, holding these points for two minutes. Apply as much pressure as you can without causing discomfort while you breathe slowly and deeply into your fear.

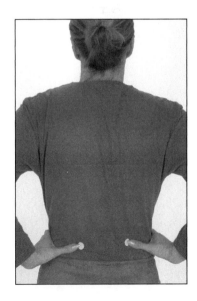

Upholding Heaven: Stand with your feet comfortably apart and your arms at your sides. Inhale, raising your arms, palms up, out to the sides and then up above your head. Interlock your fingers, with your palms facing each other. Now turn your palms inside out so that your palms face the sky. Inhale, and gently stretch farther upward, with your head tilted back. Exhale, lowering your chin to your chest, and let your arms float back down to your sides. Repeat six times.

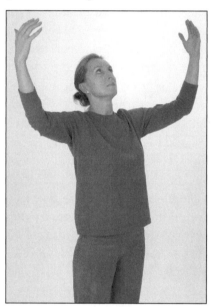 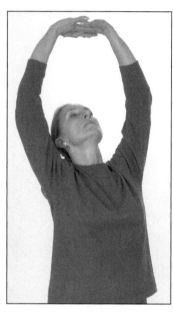

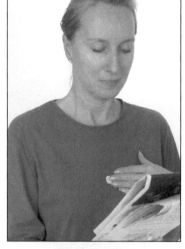

Sea of Tranquility (CV 17): Hold CV 17 on the center of your breastbone (located four finger-widths above the base of the sternum, in the indentation at the level of the heart). Pressing this calming point can open your chest, facilitate breathing, and stabilize a panic or anxiety attack.

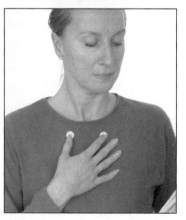

Elegant Mansion (K 27): Hold K 27 on both sides, directly below the head of your collarbones. Place your thumb on one side, and your fingertips on the other side, of the breastbone, in between the first and second ribs. Hold these chest points firmly, and breathe slowly and deeply. This can clear your throat, calm you, and counteract fear.

SELF-CARE ROUTINE
FOR FEAR & PHOBIAS

For safety, we suggest that you have a trustworthy friend or therapist present for emotional support and guidance. The following self-help exercise can be practiced sitting in a chair or lying on your back. First reflect, accept, and acknowledge how your beliefs contribute to your fear. Practice this routine regularly to deal with the roots of your fear and transform your feelings.

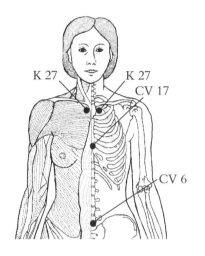

To prepare for the routine, take a towel and roll it up. Place it under your lower back, neck, or behind your knees. Experiment with different thicknesses and sizes of towels to get a comfortable pressure on both sides of the lower back. If the towel's thickness arches your back and causes pain, use a smaller towel. If the towel doesn't give you firm pressure and support, find a thicker or larger one. Placing two tennis balls inside the towel roll will boost its size and firmness greatly. Once you find a comfortable thickness, lie down on the towel roll with your eyes closed.

Step 1

Hold CV 6: Place your hands over your belly, and breathe deeply as you think back to a time when you felt fearful. Choose a frightening experience or a nightmare that you remember well from your childhood or adulthood. Breathe slowly and deeply, affirming your courage to face your fear, while placing your fingertips on CV 6 (three finger-widths below your navel). Stay in touch with your body as you recall the fearful circumstances.

If you start to feel anxious, focus on breathing slowly and deeply again, with your hands placed on CV 17 (on the center of your breastbone) to counteract any anxiety. Breathe into your courage to feel, acknowledging how fear protects you. Take a minute to explore how your fear is a healthy response when you are in danger or need to know your limits.

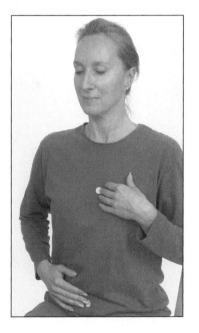

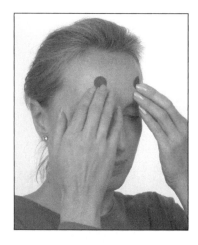

Step 2

Touch GB 14: Place your middle fingers on your forehead (GB 14, one finger-width above your eyebrows in line with the center of your pupil), using gentle touch, for one minute while breathing deeply. This point clears the mind and reprograms fearful thoughts.

Step 3

Hold K 27 with GV 24.5: First, massage your shoulders and neck for two minutes with your eyes closed. Knead any tense muscles as you focus on breathing deeply. Then lightly touch GV 24.5 (between your eyebrows) as your other hand holds K 27 firmly (in the indentations below the head of the collarbone on both sides) with your thumb and index finger. Concentrate on breathing deeply. As you inhale, breathe in the courage to face any fear or obstacle in your life. At the top of the inhalation, hold your breath for just a few seconds. Let your fear go with each complete exhalation. Continue to breathe deeply for two minutes.

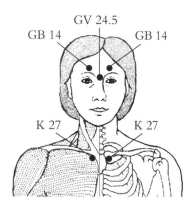

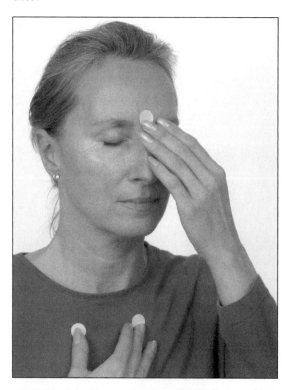

Step 4

Grasp K 6 & B 62: These points are located midway between your heel and your anklebone, on both the inner and outer ankle. Place your right foot on top of your left thigh, and grasp your ankle firmly between the anklebone and heel to press into any sore indentations. Breathe deeply as you hold these important phobia points for one minute. Then switch sides to hold the points on your left ankle. This combination helps to relieve excessive fear, stage fright, insomnia, urinary and reproductive problems, nightmares, and obsessions.

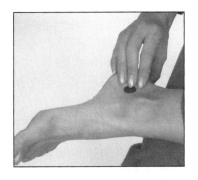

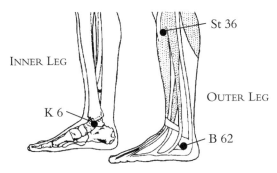

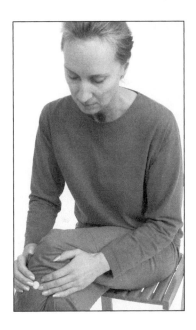

Step 5

Briskly Rub St 36: St 36 is one of the most effective acupressure points to strengthen the whole body and counteract fears and phobias. To find the point, measure four finger-widths below your kneecaps, placing your fingertips a half-inch outside the shinbone. If your fingertips are on the correct spot, you should feel a muscle flex as you move your foot up and down a few times. Use your fists to briskly rub up and down along the outside of your shinbones for one minute.

13

GRIEF

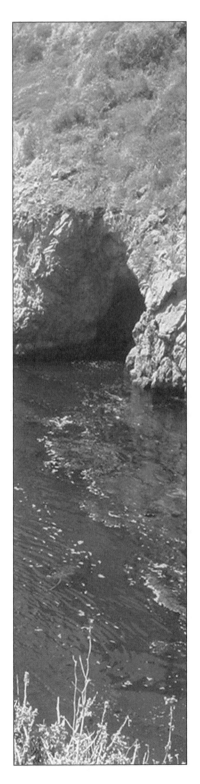

Grief is a natural response to loss, which is an inevitable aspect of life. When you lose someone or something you love, the grieving process enables you to let go and work through your conflicting feelings. For example, when someone you love dies from a serious illness that lasted a long time, you may feel a sense of relief that their suffering is over. You may also feel sadness and pain knowing you will never be together again.

Divorce is another example of a loss where one might have conflicted feelings during the grieving process. In divorce, family ties are severed, but emotional bonds remain. You may feel relieved to be free of an unhealthy marriage, but being partnerless leaves you lonely. Death and divorce are obvious reasons to grieve. Less obvious reasons are loss of a pet, a major move, retirement, miscarriage, loss of trust, or loss of a sense of spiritual connection.

Grieving people may suffer from fatigue, a weakened immune system, insomnia, disrupted sleep, and appetite imbalances. Common emotional symptoms can include anxiety attacks, depression, suicidal tendencies, numbness, sadness, and mood swings. Emotional pain and numbness from grief can cause isolation; grief can cause a person to avoid establishing new intimate relationships due to the fear of getting involved with someone they could also lose.

Everyone has different ways of experiencing loss. Grieving is an individual process; the intensity of feelings, the length of time the healing takes, and the way grief is dealt with are personal variables. Society discourages displays of the sadness and pain that are natural to the letting-go process. Many feelings of grief are labeled negative. Expressions like "Chin up, you'll find somebody else" or "Don't let the children see you crying, they'll be upset" minimize rather than facilitate the grieving process. Thus, many people have difficulty accepting and moving through grief.

Affirmations to Counteract Grief

- *I am letting go of what I expect in my life.*

- *I love myself for how deeply I feel.*

- *I am not alone; I am being taken care of.*

- *I release and let go of what I am holding on to.*

- *I trust I am being taken care of as I let go of what I loved.*

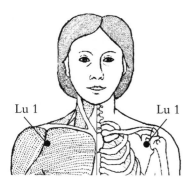

Lu 1   Lu 1

Expressing your loss and being heard are important for achieving emotional balance. During the grieving process your mind may fill up with memories, in an attempt to resolve your feelings. Resisting, ignoring, or denying this phase of the process uses up enormous quantities of energy and stresses the immune system. Give yourself enough time to reflect consciously on the past; time and reflection are the greatest healers for grief.

Sherry was in emotional shock after the suicide death of her thirty-year-old son, James. During the initial weeks of mourning she blamed herself for his death. She believed she could have prevented him from shooting himself if she spent more time with him or been a better mother. James left home at eighteen, moving away from the family. Even as a small child he spent a lot of time alone. Although Sherry often tried to reach him emotionally, James was unable to express himself or communicate his feelings. When he became more isolated in mid-life, it was not recognized as a cry for help because of James's pattern of being a loner.

For weeks Sherry couldn't sleep, eat, or interact with anyone. She isolated herself and did not communicate her feelings. The more withdrawn she became, the more her family and friends worried about her stability and mental health. They suggested and supported her to go to a psychotherapist. Eventually Sherry agreed to get some professional help. Psychotherapy opened her to healing her grief, so when a friend encouraged her to explore acupressure sessions with Beth Henning, she was ready.

Sherry's private acupressure sessions focused on her feelings of guilt about not being able to prevent James's death. Holding her upper chest and back points Lu 1, B 38, and B 15 released chest tension, feelings of guilt, and tears. Losing her child was the worst thing Sherry could imagine. She sobbed, holding on to her belly and crying out, "You're not supposed to live beyond your children!"

Sherry's grief was also accompanied by intermittent bouts of nausea, diarrhea, constipation, and fatigue. She used acupressure points to balance these physical symptoms as she continued to deal with her emotional issues and accompanying feelings. These symptoms resolved within one month, as she used the self-care routine in this chapter.

Beth's suggestion that she combine acupressure with visualization allowed Sherry to honor James in a sacred way and reunite with his spirit. She wrote poetry, drew pictures, journaled deep feelings, and practiced self-acupressure every day. She spoke about her grieving process with her family and friends, allowing them to hear and support her. Eventually she was able to participate fully in life again and reconnect with her other children. She continues to use acupressure with meditation during emotionally stressful times.

Losing full use of your body due to an accident or serious illness can also trigger feelings of deep loss and grief. Related emotions often surface long after the trauma. Car accidents, poor-quality surgeries, and severe sports injuries have caused many of Beth's clients to spend months, even years, grieving the loss of their quality of movement.

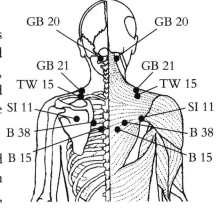

A good example is Robert, a full-time karate instructor and martial arts expert. For twenty years he spent several hours each day practicing very disciplined routines, including weight lifting, aerobics, running, and karate forms called katas.

Robert's life changed completely when he was a passenger in a severe car accident on the way to a tournament. He suffered whiplash injury and a broken right leg.

Two years after the accident he still suffered from severe neck and shoulder tension, headaches, and knee stiffness, and he remained unable to practice to his full potential. He was depressed, angry, and grieving the loss of the full use of his body when he came to Beth's office for his first acupressure session.

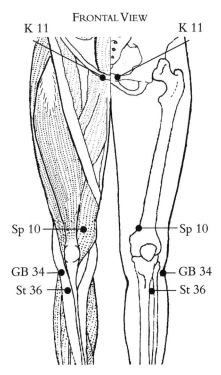

Work with the acupressure points in his shoulder-neck region (GB 21, GB 20, TW 15, and SI 11), along with deep massage for one hour, released Robert's muscular tension in the upper body and resolved his headache pain. Deep breathing with gentle stretching exercises, practicing visualization, and releasing the acupressure points on Robert's right leg and knee (Sp 10, K 11, GB 34, and St 36) helped Robert regain full use of his limb within a six-month period.

Robert depended on his physical body for his livelihood as well as his spiritual discipline. Without the healing benefits of acupressure, he might still be suffering the aftermath of his injury today.

Quick Tips for Grief

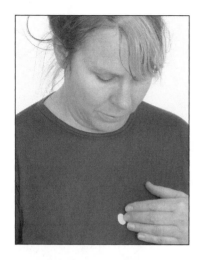

You do not have to use all of these points at one time to receive their benefits. Try one or two, when you have a few minutes to yourself. Deep breathing with acupressure opens healing energy throughout the body. For optimal results, concentrate on breathing deeply into your abdomen to cultivate overall well-being. ★

Press CV 17: The Sea of Tranquility nourishes and supports your heart during emotionally painful times. Simply bring your hands together in prayer position, placing the knuckles of your thumbs against the center of your breastbone, and breathe deeply for two minutes.

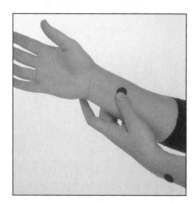

Press TW 5 with P 6: Holding the Inner and Outer Gates together will harmonize your whole body when you don't have time to practice a full routine. Hold whichever wrist feels comfortable in the center (three finger-widths above the wrist crease, on the inside and outside of the forearm). Close your eyes, and breathe deeply for two minutes.

Press P 8: Hold this emotional balancing point in the center of one palm for one minute. Then hold P 8 in your other palm.

Press Lu 1: Cross hands to hold Lu 1 three finger-widths below the outer portion of the collarbone. Close your eyes. Focus on breathing deeply, and completely relax for two minutes.

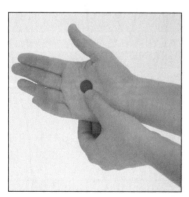

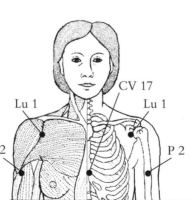

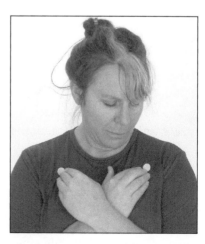

★For information on related points or topics, see Chapter 10.

SELF-CARE ROUTINE FOR GRIEF

Create a sacred healing space. Make sure you are warm and unrestricted by your clothing. Turn off the phone, turn down the lights, and concentrate on breathing slowly and deeply to discover the benefits.

Step 1

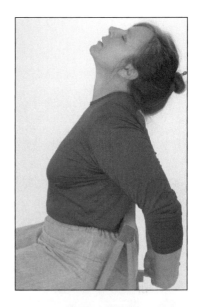

- **Back Stretch:** Sit comfortably with your spine straight and your shoulders and neck relaxed. Interlace your fingers behind your lower back with your palms facing inward. Inhale deeply as you tilt your head back, bringing your arms away from your lower back to stretch the area between your shoulder blades. Exhale as you come forward and relax. Repeat five times.

- **Leg Stretch:** Scoot up to the edge of your chair with your legs straight out in front of you. Inhale as you straighten your spine, keeping your knees straight to stretch the backs of your legs. Exhale as you slowly bring your chest down toward your knees. Inhale as you come up; exhale down. Repeat five more times.

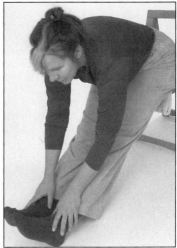

- **Lower Back Stretch:** Lie down on your back with your knees up, arms at your sides. Inhale deeply. Exhale as you slowly bring your knees to one side. Inhale as you come to center. Exhale as you slowly drop your knees to the other side. Inhale as you bring your knees back to center. Repeat from side to side as you consciously breathe deeply for two minutes.

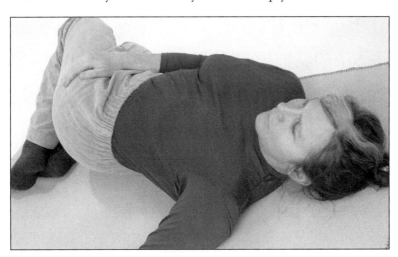

Step 2

Self-Massage: Massage and rotate your hands, wrists, and fingers. Massage and rotate your feet, ankles, and toes. Knead and squeeze your arms, shoulders, neck, and skull. Continue massaging through the torso, groin, thighs, and calves for two minutes. Then briskly brush over the surface of the areas you massaged for two more minutes.

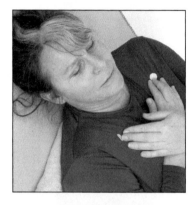

Step 3

Press Lu 1: Place a rolled-up towel underneath your mid-back. Cross your arms over your breastbone to reach the opposite Lu 1 point with the third fingertip of each hand. Take long, slow, deep breaths into your heart for two minutes. If images or tears come up, let them flow through your body.

Step 4

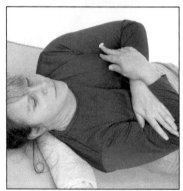

Hold P 2 with LI 11: Move your thumbs to the opposite P 2 points on the inside arm, level with the deltoid V. Use your third or fourth fingertip to press LI 11 on the end of each outside elbow crease. This point combination balances the emotions and strengthens the immune system. Breathe deeply for two minutes as you focus on what you are feeling.

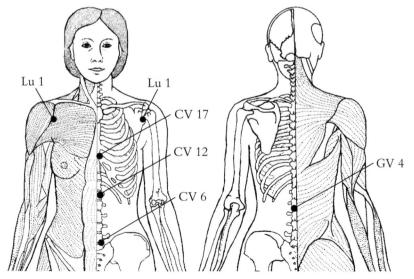

Step 5

Hold CV 12 with GV 4: Place your right hand at the center of your belly, four finger-widths down from your navel, applying moderate pressure to CV 12 with your fingertips or palm. Place your left hand underneath your back, at waist level, directly in between the lower back vertebrae (GV 4). Breathe deeply for two minutes as you inhale to receive healing energy and exhale to let go of painful emotions.

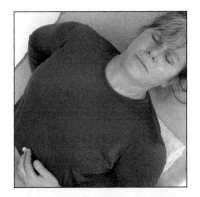

Step 6

Hold P 6 & TW 5 with CV 17: Place your left fingertips on P 6 and TW 5 (three finger-widths from the wrist crease on the inner and outer arm). Place your right palm over CV 17, to calm your heart. Breathe deeply for two minutes.

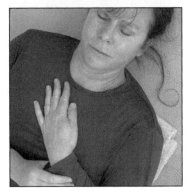

Step 7

Hold CV 6 with P 8: Place your right hand three finger-widths below your navel on CV 6. Place your left hand over your right hand, reaching the thumb to touch the center of the palm (P 8). Focus on taking long, slow, deep breaths into your belly for two minutes.

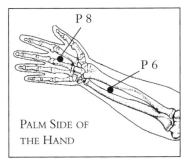

PALM SIDE OF THE HAND

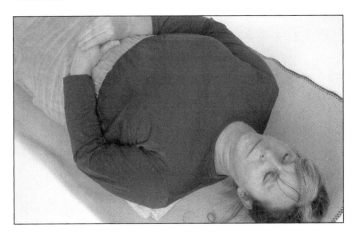

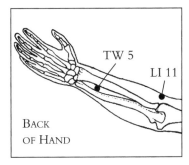

BACK OF HAND

Step 8

Deep Relaxation: Place your hands at your sides, and let yourself relax for ten minutes. Cover yourself with a blanket and rest with your eyes closed to discover the benefits.

14

GUILT & SHAME

Guilt is a degrading, painful feeling that occurs when you believe that you did something wrong or immoral. Shame is the emotional pain that comes from losing the respect of others due to perceived incompetence or improper behavior. Guilt and shame both are repressive; when these destructive emotions are continuous, serious self-doubt results, causing damage to the human spirit. The humiliation of guilt and shame makes feeling unbearable, causing emotional numbness as a protective mechanism for coping with the pain. The dishonor or disgrace associated with guilt and shame creates a negative self-image that can keep you from trusting your perceptions, intuitions, and feelings.

Guilt and shame take their toll on the internal organs. In traditional Chinese medicine, the immune system governs the kidneys, which store *chi,* the body's life energy. Being wronged, shamed, or judged in a guilty way drains the *chi,* which lowers your defenses not only psychologically but physically, weakening the immune system, which functions to defend the body from viruses and disease. The emotional pain and demeaning nature of guilt and shame also affect the Spleen meridian, which corresponds to worry and self-esteem.

The intensity of guilt and shame often stems from how you were treated as a child. Guilt and shame can be especially detrimental to a child's sense of security. The more children worry, the more they doubt themselves, which they then carry into adulthood. How often have you heard an adult tell a child, "You should be ashamed of yourself"? When parents are under stress, children are easy targets for venting frustrations. Children are often demeaned, shamed, humiliated, and abused when their caretakers are unable to cope with problems.

Adults with guilt issues tend to put the blame and shame on their children, passing on their own emotional baggage to the next generation. Parents with a poor self-image due to being

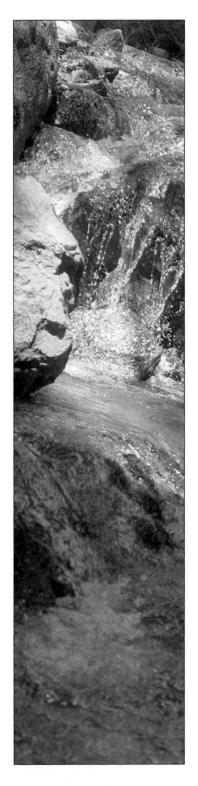

Affirmations to Counteract Guilt & Shame

- *I express my truth.*

- *I trust my instinct of what I know is right.*

- *I am grateful for who I am and release any guilt.*

- *I release the hurts of the past; all is well.*

- *My intentions are a blessing; there is no blame.*

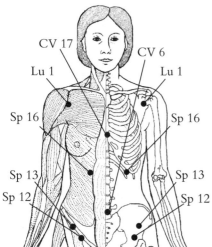

shamed in childhood may treat their children similarly, creating distrust, worry, and self-doubt. Emotionally abused children tend to have a poor self-image, excessive self-blame, and difficulty feeling their body and emotions. The trauma of guilt and shame becomes internalized as tension in the muscles of the body, numbing the emotional pain. Fortunately, acupressure combined with psychotherapy is an effective treatment for releasing hurt stored inside the body and dealing with the underlying causes.

Sara, a lesbian and middle-aged professional woman, had attempted suicide twice. Her face looked drawn from worry, stress, and tension. Her psychotherapist believed that her depression and body numbness were related to the shame and guilt she felt from her childhood. Sara had recently discontinued pain medications because the side effects outweighed the diminishing returns. The psychotherapist referred her to Beth Henning for acupressure sessions to relieve her pain and tension.

In Sara's first session, the source of her guilt and shame was revealed while Sp 12 and Sp 13 were held. Sara had been affected at an early age by her family's judgmental beliefs. Her parents were extremely prejudiced against racial minorities, women, and lesbians in their community. Sara's religious and family upbringing ingrained in her that gay and lesbian people did not have the right to live (which contributed to her later suicidal tendencies). As children, neither Sara nor her siblings dared to be different from their parents' strict expectations—yet to their parents' dismay, all of them grew up to be alcoholic, chemically dependent, or divorced.

While CV 6 was being held, Sara began to cry about her shame of being a lesbian and how her family completely rejected her. She felt deeply for her partner; they shared a powerful, nourishing love relationship. She wanted to be proud of her relationship, instead of hiding it, pretending to the world that this woman was her roommate. She mourned her inability to tell her family or friends about her lifestyle. The pressure on Lu 1 and CV 17 helped release her sadness, fears, worries, and insecurities. She cried softly for fifteen minutes as the shoulder and neck points (B 10, GB 20, and GV 16) released her chronic tension.

Sara practiced the self-care routine that follows and journaled what she wanted in her life. After four weekly sessions with Beth and daily practice of the self-acupressure routine, her numbness and tension subsided. One month later she was no longer feeling guilty about her sexuality or love relationship. She felt much more secure about herself, and her suicidal inclinations never returned.

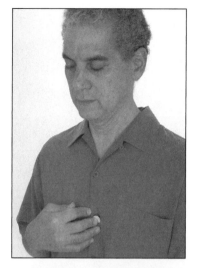

QUICK TIPS FOR GUILT & SHAME

Press CV 17, Sea of Tranquility: This point is located on the center of your breastbone, four finger-widths up from the base of the sternum. Use your fingertips to hold the indentations on the center of your breastbone. Holding CV 17 relieves nervousness, chest congestion, grief, shame, guilt, depression, hysteria, and other emotional imbalances.

Press B 23, B 47, Sea of Vitality: This point is located in the lower back, two (B 23) and four (B 47) finger-widths away from the spine at waist level. Holding these points relieves depression, shame, fatigue, exhaustion, trauma, and fear.★

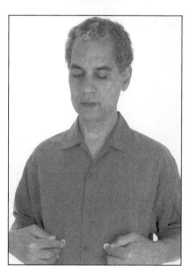

Press Sp 16, Abdominal Sorrow: This point is located below the edge of the ribcage, directly under the nipple line. Holding Sp 16 relieves indigestion, nausea, abdominal cramps, ulcer pain, worry, guilt, and blame.

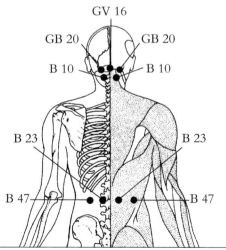

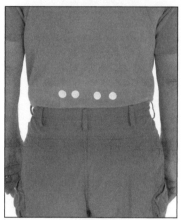

★Do not press on disintegrating disks or on a fractured or broken bone. If your back is in a weak condition, touch these points lightly. See your doctor first if you have any questions or need medical advice.

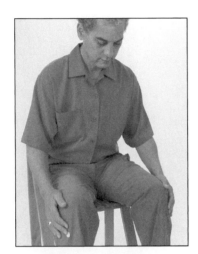

Press St 36, Three Mile: This point is located four finger-widths below the kneecap, toward the outside shinbone. Holding St 36 strengthens the whole body, tones the muscles, balances the emotions, relieves fatigue, and counteracts guilt, blame, and depression.

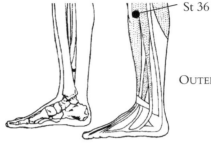

St 36

OUTER LEG

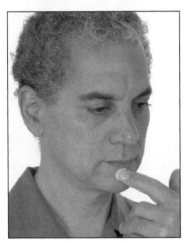

Press CV 24, Supporting Nourishment: This point is located below the center of the lower lip just above the chin. Press into the center of the lower gum. Holding CV 24 relieves allergies, throat spasms, food cravings, guilt, and obsessions; it also calms the spirit and improves concentration.

Press GV 24.5, Third Eye: This point is located between the eyebrows in the indentation where the bridge of the nose joins the forehead. Holding GV 24.5 relieves guilt, anxiety, worry, general distress, hot flashes, hay fever, sinus pain, and headache; it also balances the pituitary gland.

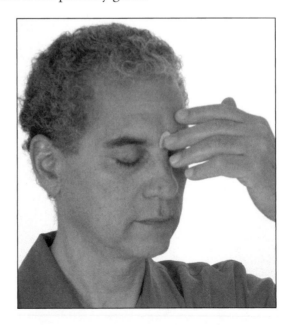

Press CV 12,★ **Center of Power:** This point is located on the midline of the body, halfway between the base of the breastbone and the belly button. Holding CV 12 relieves worry, frustration, emotional stress, self-doubt, stomach pains, abdominal spasms, and indigestion.

Press CV 6, Sea of Energy: This point is located three finger-widths below the navel. Holding it promotes emotional stability and relieves trauma, extreme fatigue, dizziness, general weakness, and confusion. Holding CV 6 also strengthens the immune system and the internal organs.

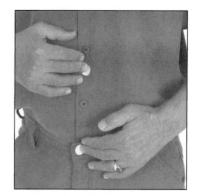

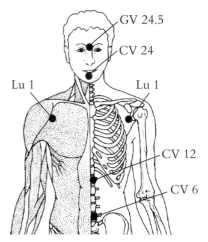

MINIROUTINE FOR GUILT & SHAME

Lie down comfortably on your back.

Step 1

Hold Lu 1: Breathe deeply into your body as you place your fingertips on your outer chest to press Lu 1, directly under the outside edge of the collarbone. Focus on any shameful memory or feeling. Affirm your safety as you breathe deeply for two minutes.

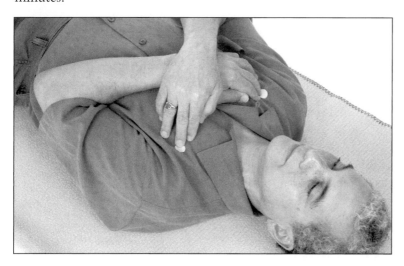

★*Caution:* Do not hold this point deeply if you have a serious illness. Hold it for no more than two minutes and only on a fairly empty stomach.

Acknowledging our wrongdoings with a genuine sense of remorse can serve to keep us on the right track in life and encourage us to rectify our mistakes when possible and take action to correct things in the future. But if we allow our regret to degenerate into excessive guilt, holding on to the memory of our past transgressions with continued self-blame and self-hatred, this serves no purpose other than to be a relentless source of self-punishment and self-induced suffering.

— His Holiness
the Dalai Lama
The Art of Happiness

Step 2

Press CV 12 & CV 17: Place your fingertips between the base of the breastbone and the navel, on CV 12.★ Gradually apply firm pressure as you breathe deeply into the point for two minutes. Ask yourself who overpowers you in your life and why. As you feel your stomach, gather an image of this person's face. As you breathe deeply, have a dialogue with this person to release any pent-up feelings. Now hold CV 17, an emotional balancing point in the center of the breastbone, and concentrate on breathing deeply for another minute.

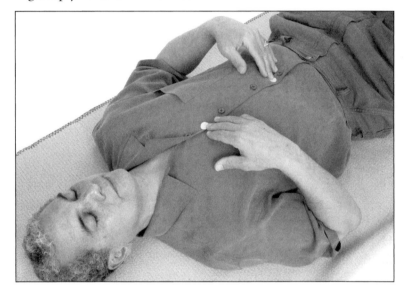

Step 3

Deep Relaxation: Allow your hands to come to your sides, and relax with your eyes closed for five to ten minutes. Before you get up, rotate your wrists and ankles and stretch like a cat. Then gradually open your eyes and sit up slowly to discover the benefits.

★*Caution:* Do not hold this point deeply if you have a serious illness. Hold it for no more than two minutes and only on a fairly empty stomach.

SELF-CARE ROUTINE
FOR GUILT & SHAME

This routine can be done in a comfortable sitting position.

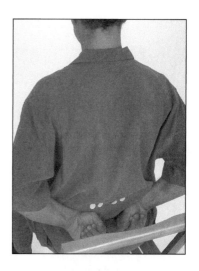

Step 1

Rub B 23 & B 47: Place the knuckles of both hands on your lower back, and rub briskly up and down to create warmth. Continue rubbing while you breathe deeply for one minute.

Step 2

Solar Plexus Meditation (Sp 16): Place your hands in front of you with your palms facing up and your fingertips facing each other. Interlace your fingers, and bring the tips of your thumbs together. Place your hands underneath the base of the ribcage, and gently press up onto Sp 16, consciously keeping your shoulders relaxed. Close your eyes, and do long, deep breathing for one minute.

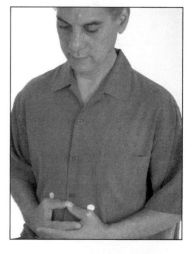

Step 3

Heart Meditation (CV 17): Place your palms together, with the backs of your thumbs against the center of your breastbone, to press CV 17. Keep your eyes closed. Breathe slowly and deeply into your heart. Make each breath longer and deeper, breathing out any stress or anxiety. After two minutes, let your hands drift down into your lap and relax. With each deep breath, allow your mind to clear.

CV 17

CV 12

Sp 16

Sp 16

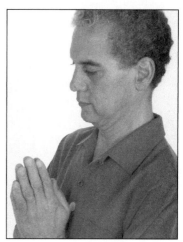

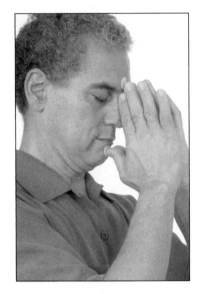

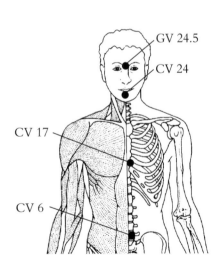

GV 24.5

CV 24

CV 17

CV 6

Step 4

Touching GV 24.5 with CV 24: Bring your palms together in front of your face, with your fingertips pointing upward. Use your middle and index fingers to lightly touch your Third Eye point (GV 24.5, between your eyebrows). Use your thumbs to touch CV 24 (between your lower lip and chin). Apply firm gentle pressure into the center of the lower gum. Make yourself comfortable, either sitting up straight or lying on your back. Close your eyes, and take several long, slow, deep breaths, using the following guided visualization to free yourself from emotional obstacles.

Explore how guilt or shame has been involved in your life… Take a few minutes to relive scenes where you were blamed or shamed… Breathe deeply as you recall snapshots or feelings of these troubling times… Breathe love into your heart as you slowly and safely allow yourself to fully be in the experience. Imagine you are face to face, speaking to the person who made you feel guilty or ashamed… Go into what happened, and continue to focus on breathing deeply throughout this visualization…

Now imagine you are on a safe path that leads to a gentle waterfall… A peaceful, calm feeling pervades you as you slowly make your way closer to the serene flowing water… Imagine how good this healing water feels as you enter the pool… Once you adjust to the water and feel refreshed, look around the waterfall, at the lush mosses and dripping ferns… Underneath the waterfall, imagine a magical space and a flat, secure rock to comfortably sit on… Feel the sound of the water gently vibrating your body… As you breathe deeply into this awesome healing environment, imagine the water rushing through your emotional wounds, washing away any shame or guilt…

Now reach your arms upward to get a good stretch… Inhale deeply, bringing in the warmth and the golden glow of sunshine into your body… Imagine the warmth of the sun radiating into your body and drying you off… As you continue to breathe deeply, explore how renewed you feel inside… Acknowledge the healing you have just accomplished as you nestle into a warm, soft robe…

Step 5

Hold CV 17 with CV 6: Place one hand on the center of your breastbone, to hold CV 17. Use your other hand to hold CV 6 (three finger-widths below your belly button). With your eyes closed, firmly press these potent points, and breathe deeply for two minutes.

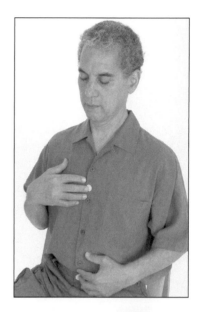

Step 6

Briskly Rub St 36: Extend your left leg straight out in front of you. Place the heel of your right foot on the St 36 point of your left leg, a few inches below the kneecap and one finger-width outside the shinbone. Briskly rub each leg for one minute, and then switch legs to rub the other side.

Step 7

Briskly Massage Your Toes: Take a minute or two to stimulate the acupressure points at the base of each toenail.

Step 8

Coming Full Cycle: Repeat Steps 1 and 2. First use the backs of your hands to briskly rub your lower back for one minute. Then relax into the Solar Plexus Meditation while taking long, deep breaths for another minute.

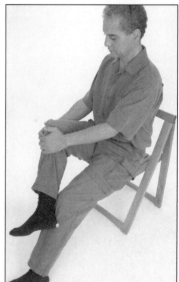

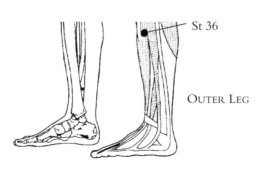

St 36

OUTER LEG

15

INCEST

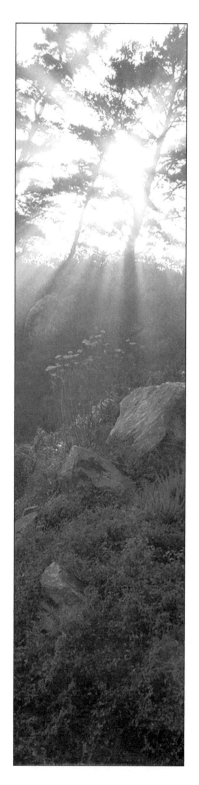

Incest is a sexual violation that causes severe emotional and physical wounds within a family. Incest is, above all, a betrayal of trust by the person or persons responsible for a child's basic needs and well-being. Most incest occurs against children, since they are vulnerable to adult manipulation and force. Perpetrators are both men and women (although the majority are men) and may include fathers and mothers, grandparents, uncles and aunts, brothers and sisters, and stepsiblings. Incest can happen once or continue for years; one-time incidents can be just as devastating as long-term episodes.

Many consider parent-child incest the greatest violation. An adult perpetrator projects his psychological imbalances onto his child, shattering the child's normal expectation of dependence and support, confusing the parent-child bond. Boundary violations, dysfunctional behavior, role confusions, shame, fear, guilt, and loss of trust all jeopardize the family's stability, causing psychological scars on all family members, often lasting a lifetime.

Incest aftereffects register for victims in the here and now and for the long term. Emotional numbness and dissociation, which we discussed in Chapter 11, are among incest's most prevalent symptoms. The child who is confused over a parental role, who receives little or no emotional support and comfort, and who lacks the wherewithal to express her confused feelings is at great risk of shutting down emotionally. Attempts to block painful feelings are completely adaptive.

Incest survivors have tremendous fears about speaking the truth of their abuse to their primary caregivers. Family members often refuse to believe them, even when the truth is staring them in the face. A child may be afraid to talk about her father's abuse with her mother, for fear of hurting her or being disbelieved. Similarly, children are afraid to tell on an older abusive sibling. In place of feeling security and trust in her family, a child may be

Affirmations for an Incest Survivor

- *I am whole;*
  I am complete.

- *I am blessed to be here*
  in the present moment.

- *As I breathe deeply,*
  I let go of being a
  victim of my past.

- *I am completely*
  released from shame,
  guilt, and fear.

- *I honor my body with*
  sacred healing touch.

- *I love myself for all that*
  I have gone through.

threatened, beaten, and even blamed for being seductive or promiscuous. Of course, many of these threats are carried out silently; the unspoken victimization and shame of sexual abuse leads to further disorientation and tremendous bewilderment.

Victims and their families keep incest buried for years. Children learn through example. During their formative years, they assimilate the lessons of their interpersonal relationships. Whatever behavior the adult role model displays becomes the child's primary understanding of reality. Children of incest are drawn to what is familiar: sexually and emotionally abusive mates.

Incest survivors often have difficulty stating their limits, since their boundaries were violated in their youth. Victims may be unconsciously attracted to situations and relationships that are familiar, even when they clearly are unhealthy and manipulative. A victim's deep and unfulfilled desire for connection and love is very attractive to users and manipulators. Charismatic and corrupt people in positions of authority (such as employers, priests, doctors, attorneys, and teachers) can find ways to take advantage of an abused person's susceptibility to power. Due to the secrecy of the relationships, offenses committed by professionals often go unreported.

The cycle of dysfunction and abuse will continue in the life of incest victims, unless they can find a way to begin the healing process and become conscious of their feelings, intentions, and behavior patterns. Fortunately, over the past two decades victims have been increasingly willing to speak up and reach out to other survivors. Education, counseling, and support groups now provide safe havens for healing.

Common Symptoms of Incest Survivors

This list covers many but not all of the symptoms that incest survivors may experience in their lifetime:

Physical Symptoms

- Insomnia
- Nightmares
- Menstrual problems
- Bulimia
- Vaginal infections
- Anorexia
- Infertility
- Ulcers

Behavioral Symptoms

- Excessive or diminished sexual activity
- Inability to make commitments
- Violence
- Difficulty with intimacy
- Difficulty building trust
- Self-blame
- Confusion
- Frequent crying

Emotional Symptoms

- Frequent crying
- Mood swings
- Depression
- Fears and phobias
- Exaggerated emotional responses
- Low or absent self-esteem
- Temper tantrums or rage reactions
- Worry and depression

There is no such thing as absolute healing. You never erase your history. The abuse happened. It affected you in profound ways. That will never change. But you can reach a place of resolution.

— Ellen Bass & Laura Davis
The Courage to Heal

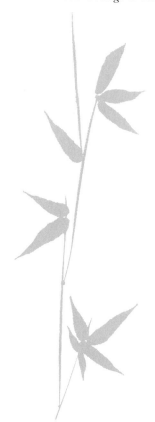

When Sandy, a middle-aged divorcée and student, came to see Beth Henning, she suffered from a bewildering number of physical and emotional symptoms such as anxiety attacks, nightmares, vaginal pain, and gastrointestinal problems. These symptoms began after she enrolled in classes at the university. Unbeknownst to Sandy, these problems were directly related to her unresolved sexual abuse at her father's hands thirty-five years earlier. Her father had had sex with Sandy from the time she was nine until she

The wounds in our emotional body are covered by the denial system, the system of lies we have created to protect those wounds. When we look at our wounds with eyes of truth, we can finally heal these wounds.

— Don Miguel Ruiz
The Mastery of Love

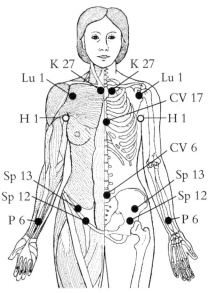

O – H 1 is in the center of the armpit.

left home at eighteen. Her mother suspected something was wrong but didn't listen when Sandy tried to tell her. As a result, Sandy grew into a quiet and reserved girl who blocked her abusive memories deep within her body.

Sandy's male art instructor was very charismatic, attractive, and charming. He often suggested she be a model in studio art classes, showing the musculature of her body, to make some extra money. Her teacher's attention and seductive tone were similar to her father's behavior during their incestuous relationship. He approached her after class one day, and they became sexually involved.

After two or three weeks of their secret relationship, Sandy had flashbacks of being in the bathtub with her father when she was a little girl. Soon afterward, other symptoms surfaced: vaginal pain, stomach pain, and anxiety attacks. Her family physician found nothing wrong, so Sandy entered therapy. With her psychotherapist's guidance, she ended the relationship with her teacher. She also realized how her body pain could be expressing her childhood emotional trauma.

After months of working on boundary issues, Sandy was encouraged to file a complaint against her teacher. This empowered her but still did not relieve her body pain. Although she had worked through the abuse images in her mind, her body continued to hold on to sensations she had felt as a child.

Sandy's psychotherapist was a client of Beth's who had successfully worked on emotional trauma in her own childhood with private sessions and acupressure self-care. She decided to refer Sandy for acupressure sessions to help release her muscle tension and body pain. She recognized the mind-body connection in deeply buried trauma cases.

Opening points in the groin area was scary for Sandy. A Pandora's box of emotion burst when she remembered her father coming into her childhood bedroom. Holding CV 6, Sp 12, and Sp 13 enabled Sandy to access buried emotions from the abuse. She screamed, "Mommy, where are you, where are you?" Holding CV 17 and P 6 helped her calm down and come back into her body safely. The emotional stress was exhausting. Deep breathing enabled her to relax, let go, and fall asleep. The cathartic experience from receiving acupressure was integrated through her psychotherapy sessions.

Unfortunately Sandy's father died before she could process with him about abusing her. Beth encouraged Sandy to use self-acupressure and journal writing, along with psychotherapy, to process her feelings. Sandy's self-care instilled trust, fostered body awareness, and supported her to reclaim her creativity and sexual energy. Sandy completely recovered from her physical symptoms and continues to use acupressure and deep breathing daily. At last report, she completed her nursing degree and was working in another state in the alternative unit of a hospital. Sandy also learned to express her feelings and needs in a healthy way and re-married.

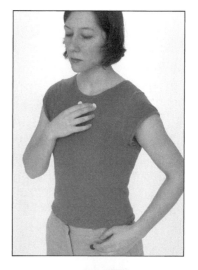

MINIROUTINE FOR
INCEST

Practice one or more of the following acupressure point combinations whenever you begin to feel numbness, insecurity, or anger.

Hold Sp 12 & Sp 13 with K 27: Hold the tighter side of the groin (Sp 12, Sp 13) with the inside edge of the collarbone (K 27) to relieve anger, numbness, or insecurity.

Hold CV 6 with Lu 1: Palm CV 6 in your lower abdomen with Lu 1 on the tightest side of your chest, to open your breathing, relieve anxiety, and revitalize your energy.

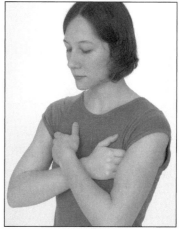

Self-Hug: Cross your arms to hold H 1 points in the center of the armpit crease, to nurture your heart. Give yourself a healing acupressure hug by placing the fingertips of your opposite hand into the opposite armpit (H 1), and breathe deeply into your heart. Close your eyes and continue to breathe deeply, affirming that the universe is a peaceful, loving place.

Hold CV 17 with CV 6: Hold these points while you breathe deeply for two minutes, to heal your heart and revitalize your spirit.

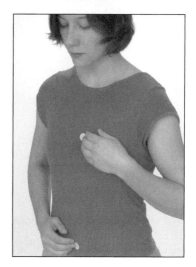

SELF-HEALING ROUTINE
FOR INCEST

*The following routine stimulates various acupressure points to open
the lower body and restore the body's energy system.*

Step 1

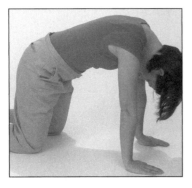

Cat-Cow Exercise: Find a comfortable place on the floor.
Place your hands on the floor in line with your shoulders and
your knees directly underneath your hips. Inhale, and arch your
spine as you bring your head up. Then drop your head down as
you exhale and relax your neck. Repeat this exercise, flexing
your spine in both directions, for one minute.

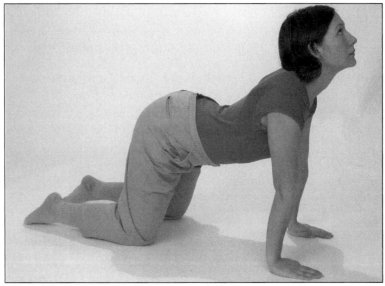

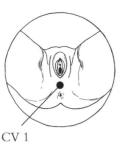

CV 1

Step 2

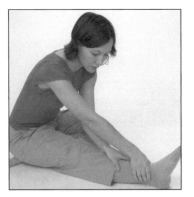

Stretch Pose: Sit on the floor with your legs in front of you.
Bend your left knee, and place your left heel on CV 1, between
your rectum and genitals. If sitting on your foot is too difficult,
simply place your left foot beside the inside of your right thigh.
Keep your right leg straight out in front of you. Inhale, and
straighten your spine. Exhale, and slowly bring your forehead toward your right knee. Continue breathing deeply, inhaling up
and exhaling down for one minute. Repeat on the other side.

Step 3

Side Rolls: Lie on your back. Bend your knees, and bring your feet in toward your buttocks. Bring your hands under your neck. Press your thumbs into GB 20 (underneath the base of your skull). Inhale deeply. Exhale as your knees come down slowly to one side. Inhale as your knees come back to center. Now exhale as your knees come down slowly on the other side. Continue twisting your body slowly from side to side for two minutes.

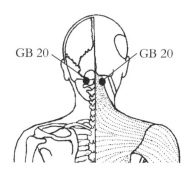

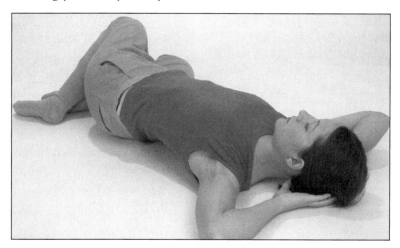

Step 4

Bridge Pose: Lie on your back with your knees bent, feet flat on the floor, and your hands resting at your sides. Bring your feet in close to your buttocks. If you can, grasp hold of your ankles. Inhale as you arch your pelvis all the way up. Breathe deeply in this position for thirty seconds. On the exhalation slowly come down.

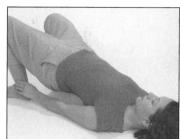

Step 5

Knee Squeeze: Bring your knees in toward your chest using your hands to hold Sp 9 (on the inside of your legs) just underneath the knee bone. Use your arm muscles to bring your knees to your chest during the exhalation. Inhale, letting the knees move away from the chest. Enjoy the movement for two minutes. Breathe deeply into your lower abdomen. Feel your lower back relax with each breath. Then let your legs come straight out and completely relax for three to five minutes.

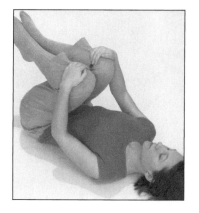

SELF-CARE ROUTINE FOR INCEST

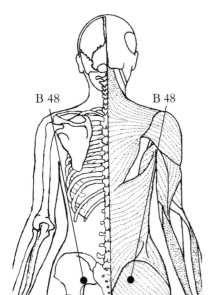

B 48   B 48

Create a healing space for yourself. You will need a towel roll and a small washcloth for this routine. Have a journal available to write down images, memories, or feelings. We suggest that you begin this routine with the Inner Child Healing Journey in Chapter 2. You do not have to do all of these steps—one or two of them can be beneficial.

Step 1

Sacrum Press: Lie on your back with a towel roll underneath your waist to support the lower back. Place your fists on B 48, two finger-widths outside the widest portion of the sacrum, at the level of your hipbone. Relax and breathe deeply, letting your weight sink onto your fists to stimulate the points. If your fists or buttocks get sore, place your hands flat underneath your buttocks with the palms down. Affirm that you are safely releasing any tension held in this area of your body. Continue for two minutes.

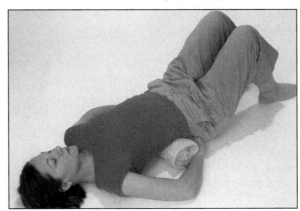

Step 2

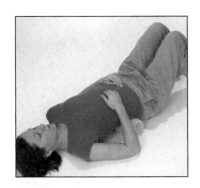

Acupressure Abdominal Massage:* Starting at CV 6 (four finger-widths below the navel), use all your fingertips to gently press into the abdominal points around your belly button. Move clockwise in a circle the size of your hand around your navel. Press and hold each position for approximately five seconds. Breathe deeply as you make three cycles around your belly, increasing the pressure gradually.

**Caution:* Do not do this step if you have just eaten or have a severe medical illness.

Allow any painful memories and images to surface as you continue to breathe deeply and massage this area. If sensations like those you felt as a child during your abuse surface, use your breath to transform your feelings. You are safe now, and no one can touch you manipulatively. If you feel anxious, move your hands to Lu 1 on the chest and breathe deeply. If you feel sad, hold your heart at the center of the breastbone (CV 17). Take care of yourself, and continue the routine when you feel ready.

Step 3

Hold Sp 12 & Sp 13: Place your fingertips on Sp 12 and Sp 13 (in the groin crease), and gradually apply firm, steady pressure onto the thick ligaments. Inhale deeply to the count of four. Then hold your breath to the count of four. Exhale slowly to the count of eight. Continue for two minutes. This exercise increases circulation through the groin and can release painful emotions associated with incest. If strong painful emotions surface, place your hands at heart level over CV 17.

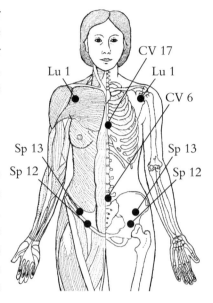

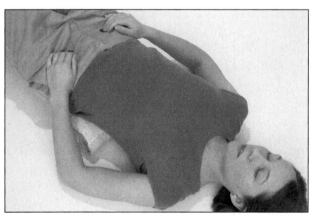

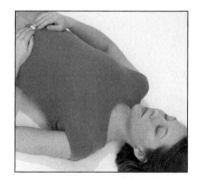

Step 4

Hold CV 6: Position a smaller rolled cloth vertically against the coccyx. Place all of your fingertips on CV 6 (three finger-widths below the belly button). Apply steady firm pressure, and breathe deeply for two minutes. Now place both palms over CV 6. Focus on breathing deeply into the healing energy flowing through your body. If you feel anxious or afraid, hold CV 17 (on the breastbone), breathing slowly and deeply.

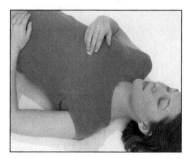

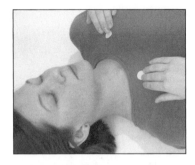

Step 5

Hold Upper Chest Points: St 13 is located below your collarbone, in the center of the chest on each side. Holding these points strengthens your sense of self-love and your personal power. Breathe deeply, affirming your courage and trust in facing the unknown. Notice feelings of resistance or tension. Focus on breathing into any pain or feelings rather than avoiding them. Pay attention to images, thoughts, and emotions that may arise, as you hold these points for two minutes.

Step 6

Self-Hug: Now hold opposite Lu 1 with the fingertips of your opposite hand. Focus on long, slow, deep breathing for two minutes. Let go of the past as you breathe slowly and deeply into your chest. Feel your heart and spirit—use your intention to clear your emotional wounds. Honor and love the child within you for the traumatic pain you have experienced.

Step 7

Palm CV 17: Place your hands (one over the other) over your breastbone, to hold your heart. Cover yourself if you feel chilled. Relax and breathe deeply for at least ten minutes to discover the benefits.

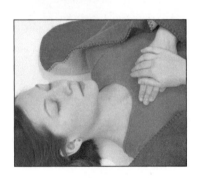

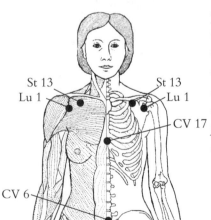

Dealing with the issues, feelings, and memories that surface through your healing process can be extremely challenging. We encourage you to create a support system, including psychotherapy, to deal with the emotional pain and memories that may surface. The rewards of staying on the path of self-healing are empowering for living a more balanced life. For greater effectiveness, give your self-acupressure quality time and commitment. Shift your attention to your willingness to heal. By practicing the exercises given here, you are taking significant steps to heal yourself.

St 13
Lu 1
St 13
Lu 1
CV 17
CV 6

16
JEALOUSY & RESENTMENT

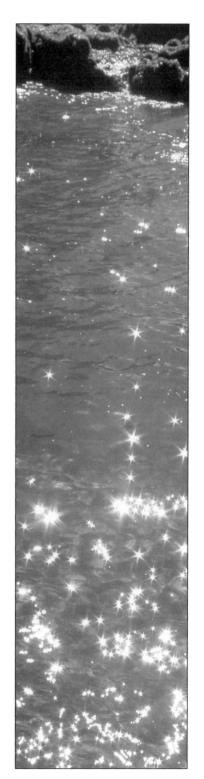

W hen you have shared the deepest, most cherished parts of yourself with someone who cheats on you and otherwise turns away from you, who doesn't listen to you or treat you with respect, jealousy rears its head. Resentment, disappointment, and bitterness usually follow in its wake, along with anger, fear, panic, anxiety, humiliation, sadness, or depression.

Jealousy also opens the door to obsessing over unresolved memories and issues from the past. Jealous feelings may cause muscle tension in the chest, neck, shoulders, and upper back. Using acupressure and the self-care routines in this chapter can help you to relax tense areas of the upper body, redirect your anger, and calm reactive feelings.

Elizabeth was a married, middle-aged professional mother of two who suffered from chronic upper body and neck pain, TMJ with associated tooth pain, moodiness, and general negativity. Medication and psychotherapy temporarily resolved her problems. After reading a magazine article that talked about the benefits of acupressure and massage for body pain and stress, she sought alternative care.

Elizabeth's husband was an instructor and often out of town, presenting workshops and speeches throughout the year. Many of his business and teaching associates were women. Although Elizabeth trusted him, she feared that he would leave their relationship for something better. Despite his attempts to appease her jealousy, she became overcome with insecurity. Her body pain and mood swings were caused by fantasies of being abandoned and betrayed by the man she loved.

Affirmations to Counteract Jealousy & Resentment

- *I let go of jealousy and resentment; holding on doesn't serve me anymore.*

- *As I breathe deeply, I open to the infinite possibilities of love and life.*

- *I attract trusting and loving relationships.*

- *I choose to be mindful and express my feelings.*

- *Each deep breath fills me with peace and good energy.*

During her first acupressure session, Elizabeth was encouraged to feel the jealousy she stored in her body. She clenched her fists, tightened her jaw, and pounded on the table. Holding St 3 and St 6 released her jaw tension. She learned to use these points daily in a self-care routine, which completely resolved her tooth and TMJ pain.

Holding CV 6, in the lower belly, released Elizabeth's anger and resentment toward her husband. As she let go of her resentment, she discovered valuable insights about her fears of being unlovable. Her fear of rejection was at the core of her pain. Moving through these emotional layers in her first session was transformational in resolving this issue and healing her physical symptoms. Holding Letting Go (Lu 1) and Elegant Mansion (K 27) released her sadness and grief for the loss her resentment incurred. Acupressure stabilized her emotions, gave her inner strength, and increased her awareness of her insecurities.

Elizabeth's greatest weakness thus became an ally for growth and empowerment. Once she became aware of the nature of her insecurities, she was able to transform them. Awareness is an important first step in emotional healing.

Three weeks of self-care resolved Elizabeth's physical symptoms. Releasing her jaw tension opened up her throat and her ability to speak clearly and intimately with her husband about her fears. Communication and trust restored her heart. Fortunately her husband was able to receive this communication in a constructive, loving way. Instead of holding on to jealousy, Elizabeth was able to express and resolve her feelings. She learned to use the time her husband was away for self-nourishment and growth in regular counseling sessions, exercise, self-acupressure, and journaling. These activities would also allow her to counteract the negative feelings and emotional unease that occasionally crossed her mind.

In traditional Chinese medicine, anger and resentment are governed by the Liver meridian. Thus a person with repressed anger may eventually develop problems associated with the liver. Similarly, a person who has a congested, overtaxed liver may easily become angry and resentful. On the other hand, if the liver is in good condition, a person will be able to express anger assertively in a healthy, constructive way.

SUGGESTIONS FOR BALANCING
JEALOUSY & RESENTMENT

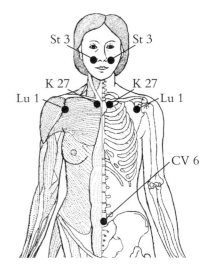

- **Increase Whole Grains:** Whole grains such as barley, wheat germ, millet, and brown rice are calming and can contribute to discharging negative emotions. In addition, well-cooked whole grains nourish the digestive system.

- **Increase Protein:** Emotional instability lessens when good-quality protein is added to the diet. Increasing tofu, fish, and beans and limiting animal products can be beneficial to your diet when you're under emotional stress. Too much animal protein, in the form of red meat and dairy foods, can overstimulate the liver and exacerbate feelings of jealousy, anger, and resentment.

- **Eliminate Stimulants:** Avoid caffeine, tobacco, recreational drugs, alcohol, excessive sex, hot spices, and overeating in general. Instead drink water with lemon at room temperature. In addition, eat mild foods and herbs.

- **Eat Regularly:** Avoid eating late at night and especially before sleeping. Jealousy and resentment often disturb sleep patterns. Overeating before bedtime exacerbates these emotions and causes nightmares.

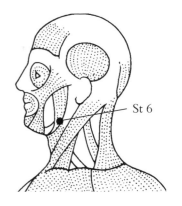

- **Think Positively:** Spend time each day affirming your intention. Tell yourself that you are lovable and capable of creating relationships that are healthy and trustworthy. Prayer, deep breathing exercises, and meditation can facilitate positive spiritual awareness.

- **Do Aerobic Exercise:** Running, swimming, biking, cross-country skiing, and climbing hills are excellent ways to vent and keep rage and resentment from getting blocked inside your body.

- **Seek Mental & Emotional Support:** Counseling, psychotherapy, talking to a good friend, and journal writing can enable you to process your issues and feelings. Calm your mind, nurture your heart, and become conscious of your needs to counteract jealousy.

- **Participation in Spiritual Activities:** Meditation, self-acupressure, yoga, tai chi, religious services, prayer, and other spiritual practices can support you in transforming your jealousy and resentment.

- **Increase Flexibility:** Stretch for five minutes three times per day. Gently stretch the insides of your legs and the sides of your body, to release the emotional toxins associated with jealousy and resentment. Stretching also benefits the liver. Habitual stretching keeps the mind and body flexible.

QUICK TIPS FOR
JEALOUSY & RESENTMENT

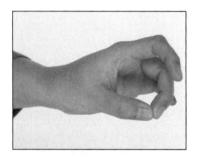

The following finger positions can be effective for releasing jealousy and anger when you don't have time to do a full routine. Lightly touching specific fingers together comes from an ancient yogic tradition called mudras. *You do not have to use all of these positions to gain benefits—using one or two when you have a free hand can be beneficial. Choose from the following positions, or create your own by combining fingers related to specific emotional issues.*

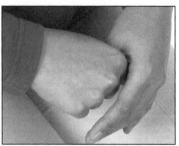

Thumb with Middle Finger: Close your eyes, and breathe deeply as you touch the tip of your thumb to the middle fingertip. Hold this hand position for two minutes. The thumb represents willpower; the middle finger governs mental and emotional well-being. Practice with both hands at once or one hand at a time.

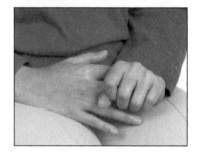

Thumb: Grasp the thumb of the opposite hand. Breathe deeply, and hold for two minutes. This position enhances your breathing and supports you in letting go of whatever you need to release.

Middle Finger: The middle finger affects your mental-emotional balance and protects your emotional well-being. By holding the middle finger with the opposite hand, you can calm your inner and outer world. Breathe deeply and hold for two minutes.

SELF-CARE ROUTINE FOR
JEALOUSY & RESENTMENT

Jealousy and resentment can frequently involve the underlying emotions of anger and rage. The following self-care routine discharges anger while facilitating deep healing and conscious awareness. For the best results, focus on breathing slowly and deeply. Be sure to seek help from a counselor, or therapist, or a trustworthy, emotionally stable friend if your anger and rage feel too big to handle alone.

We suggest you practice this routine in a private space where you will be uninterrupted and free to make sound. Use pillows or other soft objects to pound and let out your anger. A picture or other item that triggers your resentment can be helpful. Use soft lighting. You will need a towel, a mat, and a light blanket or sheet to cover you.

Allow yourself a fixed amount of time to focus on the source of your rage, resentment, or jealousy. Accept and love yourself for what you are going through. Breathe deeply into your heart while experiencing these emotions. Practicing these exercises can decrease the amount of time you spend in obsessive thought, release negative emotions, and increase your overall ability to heal. ★

Once the work of resolving resentments is under way, the choices for diet and other lifestyle factors should fall into place. Without this work, one tends to eat and live in ways that support the old, unresolved patterns.

— Paul Pitchford
Healing with Whole Foods

Step 1

Focus on Object: Begin by focusing on the picture or other object that triggers your resentment. Breathe deeply, and allow your body to feel without judging or blocking your emotions.

• **Build Emotions:** Clench both fists tightly and inhale, breathing in the courage to feel your jealousy and resentment. Let your emotions build.

★For additional assistance with jealousy and resentment, see Chapters 7 and 17. If these routines don't facilitate release of your negative emotions after a few weeks of daily practice, seek professional support.

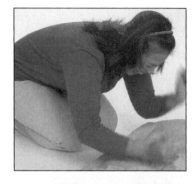

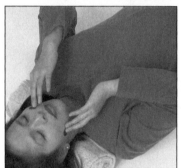

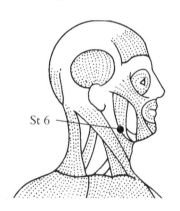

- **Release Sound:** As you exhale, allow a sound, like a deep sigh, to come out. Sound can release and transform jealousy and resentment. Continue to deepen your breath. Increase the volume of your sound as you pound the pillows. If your mind wanders, use the photograph or object to refocus. Allow your body to express itself through your pounding, sounds, and tears. After several minutes, if you feel you need more time to release your agitation, continue this exercise for another five minutes.

Lie comfortably on your back for the next step. If you have lower back pain, use a couple of pillows under your knees. Roll up a towel and place it at the base of your spine at waist level. Adjust the towel and make yourself comfortable.

Step 2

Hold St 3 & the Jaw (St 6): Breathe deeply and fully as you make firm contact with St 3 (under your cheekbone) and St 6 (in the center of your jaw muscles). Allow yourself time to explore, feel, and release this area. These points release tension associated with jealousy. Continue holding these points for two minutes as you breathe deeply into your lower abdomen.

Step 3

Press K 27: Use your fingertips to press K 27 (underneath the inside head of the collarbone, in the indentation between your first and second ribs). Take full, deep breaths, making firm contact for two minutes, to revitalize your body.

St 6 —

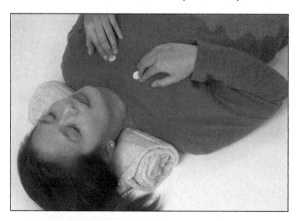

Step 4

Palm CV 6 & CV 12: Place the palm of your right hand over your mid-diaphragm over CV 12, and the palm of your left hand over your lower abdomen three fingers below your belly button (CV 6). Holding these areas enhances your self-image, sense of personal power, and ability to build healing energy. Breathe deeply into your hands. Continue for two minutes.

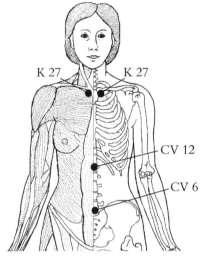

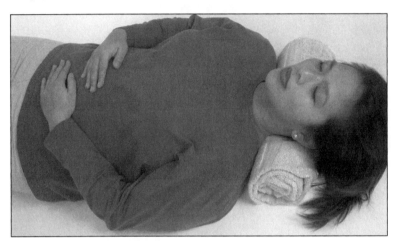

Step 5

Deep Relaxation: Place your hands at your sides. Cover yourself with a blanket or sheet, and begin long, slow, deep breaths. Breathe in love for yourself. Relax and discover the benefits for five to ten minutes.

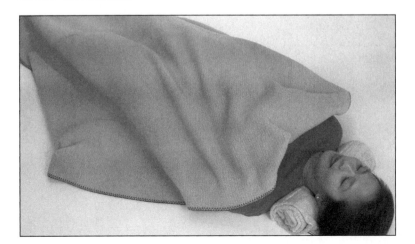

17

MOOD SWINGS

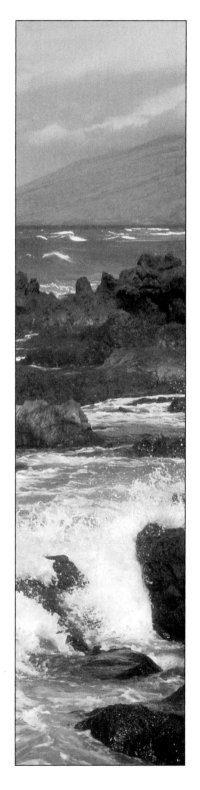

Bonnie, a long-term client of Michael Gach, had a sweet, likable personality. People were often drawn to help her because of her adorable nature. But she suffered from mood swings. Since childhood her life was a series of dramas, a roller-coaster ride of extreme highs and lows. She had difficulty coping with everyday stress and was often overwhelmed.

Bonnie's need for love, approval, and recognition contributed to her mood swings. As a child, she did not receive the attention that she needed from her parents, which consequently affected her self-image. Although Bonnie was an attractive young woman, she doubted herself and worried constantly. Her mood swings and craving for affection contributed to her codependent relationships and emotional instability.

Bonnie's strong sugar cravings were a major culprit in creating her instability. Each morning she would wake up negative, grumpy, and irritable. Then she would eat her regular breakfast of pastries, coffee, and a large glass of fruit juice.

Acupressure points for balancing instability and mood swings were selected for Bonnie's self-care program. She worked with these points for six months to battle her sweet cravings. When she made the commitment to stop eating sugar, her mood swings and irritability changed significantly. Once she became aware of her destructive beliefs about not being good enough and used the acupressure points, she made steady progress toward regaining balance. The safety of acupressure's treatment touch supported Bonnie in renewing her connection with her body, which shifted her attitudes and heightened her self-image.

We found that mood swings and bipolar disorder responded well to using acupressure, deep breathing, daily aerobic exercise, and dietary considerations. Increased effectiveness results from combining these complementary self-treatment practices with psychotherapy, especially for severe cases of bipolar disorder.

Affirmations to Counteract Mood Swings

- *I love, accept, and respect myself.*

- *I am strong enough to say no to eating sweets.*

- *I make wise, healthy choices that support my well-being.*

- *I believe in myself and live joyfully.*

DIETARY CONSIDERATIONS

Sugar is a defeating ingredient in many people's lives. In its various forms it weakens many body functions, especially the immune system, and causes emotional instability. To counteract mood swings, eliminate all foods that contain sugar, including brown sugar, cane sugar, cane juice, date sugar, corn syrup, maple syrup, honey, and fructose. Reduce the intake of all fruits and juices, except for apples and pears. These foods dilute your blood and can cause hypersensitivity, irritability, and overwhelming feelings. Also limit eating ice-cold foods and drinks. (See Chapter 26 for more information.)

Cut out sugar by starting with small steps. First minimize your intake of sugar, and avoid refined sugars and high-fructose corn syrup. Each day reduce your sugar intake a little more. Try using fruit-sweetened products available in health food stores instead of refined sugar and honey. Gradually wean yourself off sugar completely for at least three months; afterward notice your emotional stability. Here are suggestions to counteract sweet cravings:

- **Licorice root**—the herb, not the candy—has a sweet taste. Sucking on it can curtail sugar cravings.

- **Use stevia** (found in most health food stores) in liquid or powder form as a sugar substitute. Stevia leaf balances blood glucose and maintains healthy blood pressure. It has been used for hundreds of years in South America.

- **Eat a little bit of fruit** instead of refined sugar.

- **Eat more steamed vegetables** such as carrots, beets, zucchini, squash, and corn. Steam these vegetables whole to retain their sweet, nutritious juices and strengthen your condition.

- **Baked yams and baked apples** are naturally sweet and can curb your desire for sugar.

- **Vigorous aerobic exercise** for at least twenty minutes makes you sweat, which detoxifies your body and rebalances your metabolism to counteract sweet cravings.★

★For more information about mood swings, see Chapters 10, 24, and 26.

SPECIAL POINTS FOR
MOOD SWINGS

Hold any of the following points for one to three minutes each, to balance emotional instability and contribute to strengthening the body's physical constitution.

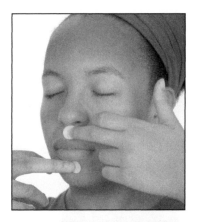

Press CV 24 & GV 26: Holding these points (located on the center of the lower and upper gums) enhances mental clarity, restores emotional stability, and counteracts sugar cravings.

Press K 27: Holding this point (located in the hollows below the head of the collarbone, next to the breastbone) relieves anxiety, depression, chest congestion, and breathing difficulties.

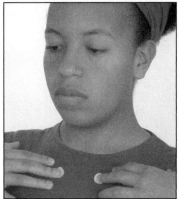

Press Sp 16: Holding this point (located on the lower edge of the ribcage, four finger-widths out from the center of the body) relieves appetite imbalances, sugar cravings, mood swings, worry, and self-doubt.

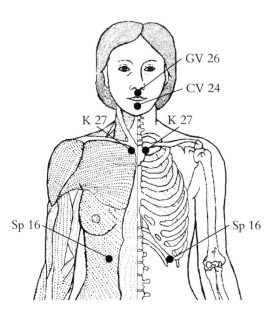

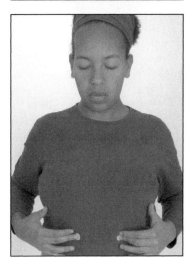

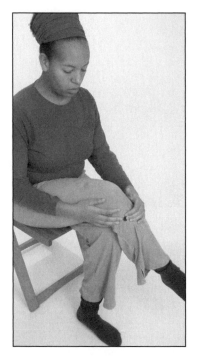

Press St 36: Holding this point (located four finger-widths below the kneecap, one finger-width to the outside of the shinbone) fortifies the body with energy, tones the muscles, and counteracts sugar cravings. Press this point regularly if you feel emotionally unstable or have mood swings.

Press Sp 3: Holding this point (located on the upper arch, behind the ball of the foot) regulates blood sugar levels.

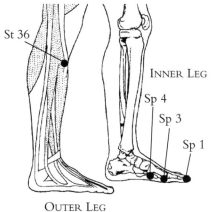

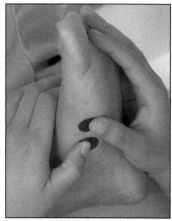

Press Sp 4: Holding this point (located on the middle of the arch, one thumb-width from the ball of the foot) counteracts sugar cravings.

Press Lv 3: Holding this point (located on the top of the foot, in the valley between the bones of the big toe and second toe) balances the liver and relieves confusion as well as depressing mood swings.

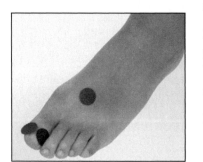

Press Sp 1 & Lv 1: Holding these points (located at the base of the large toenail) stimulates the pituitary, the master endocrine gland.

QUICK TIPS FOR WHEN LIFE'S OVERWHELMING

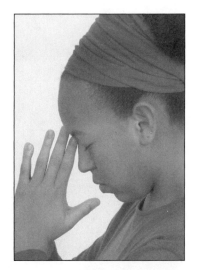

Press GV 24.5: Sit with your spine straight, eyes closed, and chin tilted down slightly. Bring your palms together, and use your middle and index fingertips to lightly touch the Third Eye point (GV 24.5) between your eyebrows. Take long, slow, deep breaths for two minutes as you visualize yourself going to a place that makes you feel calm, restful, and safe—a place where you can trust yourself.

Press CV 17: Keeping your palms together, use the back of your thumbs against your breastbone to press the Sea of Tranquility point (CV 17) firmly, at the level of your heart. Keep your eyes closed, and concentrate on breathing slow, even, deep breaths into your heart to completely dispel the overwhelming feelings. Make each breath longer and deeper. Breathe out any tension you may feel, allowing each deep breath to clear your mind.

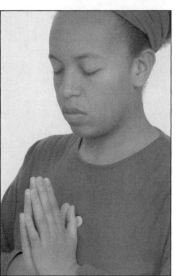

Press CV 6: Place your fingertips three finger-widths directly below the belly button, and gradually press into the center of your lower abdomen. Sit back comfortably in a chair with your spine straight and your shoulders relaxed. Close your eyes, press firmly into this point, and breathe deeply for two minutes to stabilize your emotions and strengthen your internal organs.

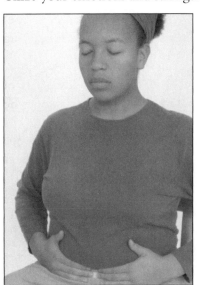

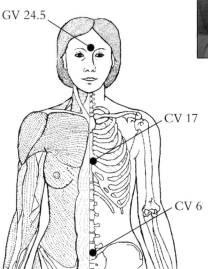

GV 24.5

CV 17

CV 6

QUICK TIPS FOR MOOD SWINGS

Sit comfortably to work on these powerful points for relieving mood swings. You do not have to use all of them; one or two alone can be beneficial.

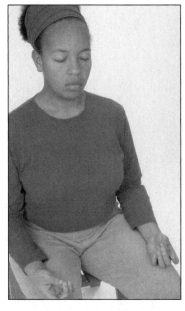

Rub St 36: Place your knuckles on St 36 (four finger-widths below your kneecap, a half-inch outside the shinbone). With your right fist on the outside of your right leg and your left fist on the outside of your left leg, briskly rub up and down beside the shinbone for one minute. This is very effective for counteracting mood swings.

Index & Middle Fingers: Hold your index and middle fingers firmly for a minute. Close your eyes, and breathe deeply to oxygenate your blood. Then switch to hold the fingers on your other hand firmly for another minute, as you breathe deeply and relax. This simple finger exercise balances your emotions, harmonizes mood swings, and calms your spirit.

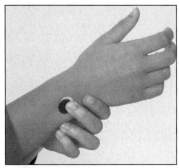

Hold TW 5 with P 6: Hold these points (located three finger-widths below the wrist crease, on the inner and outer wrists) for two minutes. Quiet your mind and focus on breathing deeply. Use this simple exercise to relieve mood swings.

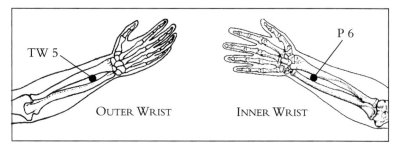

TW 5   OUTER WRIST   P 6   INNER WRIST

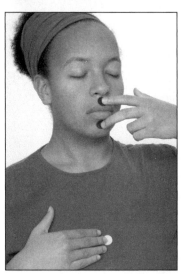

Hold CV 17 with CV 24 & GV 26: Place all of the fingertips of your left hand on CV 17 (on the center of your breastbone in the indentations at heart level). Use your right hand to press GV 26 and CV 24 simultaneously. Place your index finger on GV 26 (between the base of the nose and the upper lip). Use your middle finger on CV 24 (between your lower lip and your chin). Press deeply enough to apply firm pressure on your upper and lower gums for two minutes.

SELF-CARE ROUTINE FOR
MOOD SWINGS

The following routine can help you manage sugar cravings, worry, irritability, stress, and mood swings. It can be practiced sitting in a chair or lying on your back. Concentrate on breathing deeply.

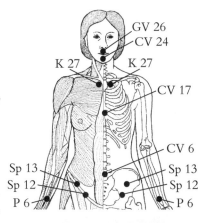

Step 1

Back Press: Roll up a towel, and place it under your lower mid-back area. Keep it there as long as it's comfortable. Breathe deeply while doing the following steps.

Step 2

Hold K 27 with CV 6: Place your thumb and middle fingers on K 27 (in the hollows directly below the inner protrusions of the collarbone). Place the fingertips of your other hand on CV 6 (in the center of your lower abdomen, between your belly button and your pubic bone). Take long, deep breaths as you hold these points for two minutes.

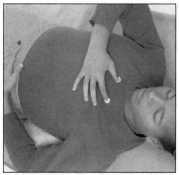

Step 3

Hold Sp 12 & Sp 13: Hold these points (located in the pelvic area, on the middle of the crease where the leg joins the trunk of your body). Firmly press the cordlike ligament just above this crease for two minutes.

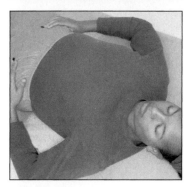

Variation (Locust Pose): If you are able to lie down on your stomach, place your fists underneath your groin, where your thigh meets the trunk of your body. Place your forehead or chin, whichever is more comfortable, on the floor. Bring your feet together; inhale, and raise your feet up with your thighs off the ground. Breathe deeply into your belly with your legs up for thirty seconds. Then slowly come down, and bring your hands by your sides. Turn your head to one side, adjust your body comfortably, and completely relax for two minutes.

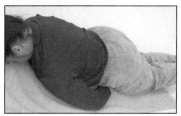

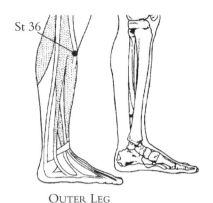

St 36

OUTER LEG

Step 4

Rub St 36 with Your Heel: Sit or lie on your back. Extend your left leg straight out. Bend your right leg, and place your right heel on St 36 (located on the outside of your left leg, four finger-widths below the bottom of your kneecap). Briskly rub your heel up and down on the outside of your shinbone. After one minute, switch and do the other side for another minute.

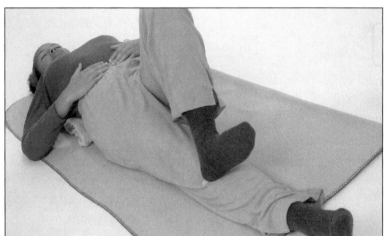

Step 5

Firmly Rub Lv 3: Place your right heel on Lv 3 (at the top of your left foot, at the junction between the large and second toes). Use your heel to rub this important liver point for one minute. Repeat on the other side.

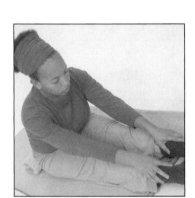

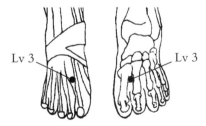

Lv 3   Lv 3

Step 6

Leg Stretch: Reach forward to hold your ankles or large toes for one minute. Keep your legs straight enough to get a gentle stretch. After a couple of deep breaths, gently shake out your legs and relax quietly with your eyes closed for several minutes.

18

SEXUAL ABUSE

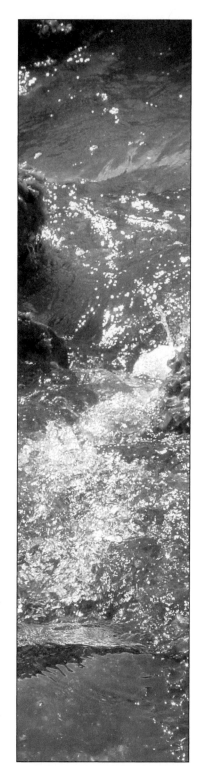

Nancy, one of Beth Henning's acupressure clients, described how her sexual healing occurred: "While the points in my groin (Sp 12, Sp 13) were pressed, I remembered being held down and sexually abused. I was a little girl when I was sexually molested. At that time, I decided I needed to be passive in order to survive. I was helpless, suppressed, pinned down against a wall. The harder I tried to get away, the worse it got. I decided to be still and pretend like nothing was happening. The fear of responding and making things worse made me hold my breath. I became invisible in order to stay alive. My childhood experience was so traumatic that I continued to feel invisible and victimized in adult life.

"Holding points on myself and having acupressure sessions with Beth enabled me to release stress and trauma. By reexperiencing the abuse, I was able to release negative feelings I'd held in my body for years. As a result, I learned that I do not need to pretend to be helpless in my life. Acupressure helped me release the roots of my powerlessness by becoming self-reliant. Regaining a sense of my own body and trusting myself have been vital in healing my possibilities for intimacy."

Nancy responded well to acupressure right away; in her first session the safe touch enabled her to open up and feel her body for the first time in many years. After several sessions with Beth and acupressure self-care, Nancy was able to release the roots of her powerlessness and accept her adult self. She continued to receive monthly acupressure sessions for a year, as ongoing support to nurture her renewed sense of self and integrate her healing.

Marlene, another client of Beth's, was sexually abused for most of her young life. At forty she suffered from chronic gynecological problems and depression. Doctors prescribed long lists of medications for her multitude of symptoms, which included insomnia and vaginal pain. Marlene's emotional and physical pain

Affirmations for Sexual Healing

- *I trust that I am being taken care of.*

- *I am loved unconditionally.*

- *My body is well, sacred, and intact.*

- *I am a vessel of love, harmony, and aliveness.*

- *I completely forgive and release any past emotional pain.*

was directly related to her sexual abuse. She became conscious of this when her own daughter turned ten; this was the age in Marlene's childhood when the sexual abuse increased and became more violent.

When Marlene's memories surfaced, she felt a sharp pain in the genital area. Acupressure enabled her to recognize the interrelationship between her emotions and her physical pain. While Beth held acupressure points on her body, strong feelings surfaced in Marlene, accompanied by vivid images of her sexual abuse. These images were the by-product of discharging her emotions. Tears flooded her eyes like a rolling river; as memories consumed her mind, severe abdominal cramping took over. Often she would get nauseous in a session. Acupressure, along with deep breathing, finally released the physical ailments and emotional pain she had held inside from her sexual abuse.

Marlene's attraction to asexual men had enabled her to avoid feelings of shame and guilt about her own sexuality. She had learned to equate sex with pain, not pleasure. Eventually she released these feelings through acupressure and was able to enjoy a healthy sexual relationship. After receiving a series of acupressure sessions over a five-month period, she developed a sense of aliveness and creativity.

Sexual abuse can create emotional wounds, fear, and distress that block the flow of energy, positive sexual feelings, and intimacy. A huge range of emotions, varying from emotional and bodily numbness to hypersensitive feelings and even disgust at another person's touch, are direct results of the deep shame of sexual abuse, whether the events occurred during childhood, in adolescence, or in adulthood. Abuse victims may be hypersensitive to physical touch as well as what people say and how they act.

Sexual abuse often causes psychological, physical, social, and sexual trauma in various combinations. Both sexual abuse and sexual trauma can result in psychological aftereffects such as denial, repression, avoidance of places or objects that induce memories of the traumatic incident, fears, panic attacks, feelings that something is missing or not right, depression, alcohol and substance abuse, suicidal thoughts, recurring and intrusive thoughts and dreams about the traumatic incident, nonspecific health problems, eating disorders, sexual avoidance, and relationship problems.

Abuse survivors may appear overly sensitive to physical contact because for them the sensuality of touch can trigger memories of the traumatic experience that feel as real as if they were happening again, which is called reexperiencing. Shameful feelings, guilt, and fears can surface, shutting out intimacy and love. When these feelings are reexperienced in a safe environment, however, the survivor has an opportunity to consciously express and release the emotional pain long held within the body.

INNER CHILD SEXUAL HEALING

You can heal your sexuality further by exploring early childhood memories and feelings related to sexual trauma and abuse. Inner child work is invaluable for deepening acupressure's emotional balancing process, especially for healing sexual wounds. (See the Inner Child Healing Journey at the end of Chapter 2.)

Profound emotional and sexual healing can occur if you cultivate a relationship with the part of yourself that was once a child. This child within you, your inner child, knows your emotional needs. Communicating with your inner child about traumatic events can be surprisingly therapeutic. Many inner child journeys are needed to heal emotional pain from sexual abuse.

Dealing with incest and sexual abuse often brings up resistance, shame, and confusion. These feelings, along with fuzzy memories of what happened, make it difficult to access traumatic experiences. You may doubt the trauma even happened. Recalling memories may be painful and create resistance. In addition, your memory and images of the trauma may be distant and obscure. The following story illustrates how acupressure can heal an emotional trauma through visual imagery of the inner child.

One night, Joan and her husband, a prominent accountant, attended a large party. As they were drinking martinis with a "new friend," her husband excused himself to go to the bathroom. The "new friend" evidently drugged Joan's drink! He convincingly said, "I am going to take you to a very special place, and your

The emotions related to abuse can be overwhelming and often conflicting. We may feel both intense longing and betrayal, with a simultaneous urge to both reach out and withdraw. We may feel expansive anger and contracting fear at the same time. We may feel strong emotions at some times and numbness at others.

— Anodea Judith
Eastern Body Western Mind

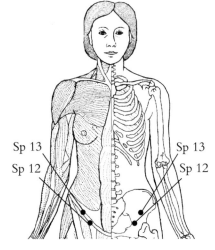

Sp 13
Sp 12

Sp 13
Sp 12

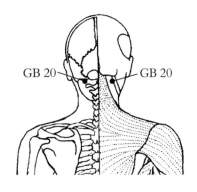

GB 20

GB 20

husband will meet us later." She felt something wasn't quite right, but the drug distorted her boundaries and perceptions, completely debilitating her. He entrapped her upstairs in an abandoned apartment building for the entire night, where he raped her; she felt as helpless as a little girl.

Several months after this tragic incident, Joan began acupressure therapy with Michael Gach to heal her emotional wounds. Acupressure enabled her to be extraordinarily visual and reexperience clearly the sexual abuse that had occurred. She remembered the man taking off her red dancing shoes and also saw flashbacks of her own bedroom when she was a little girl. The drug numbed her adult self and left her vulnerable, like an unprotected child. In her first session Joan was able to release some of her guilt for not setting her boundaries.

After holding the points between her shoulder blades and underneath her ribcage, Michael worked on her chest points and encouraged her to breathe deeply. She realized how the child within her felt hurt, used, betrayed, and abandoned. She reexperienced herself as a little girl curled up in a ball in the darkest corner of the room she was trapped in, with her head hanging forward, crying.

There was a split between Joan's inner child and her adult self. Her adult self still felt shame and guilt. Michael encouraged her adult self to talk to her inner child and bridge the gap. Her muscles were tense; her points would not release. Her images were strong and vivid, clearly showing the little girl's resistance, anger, and resentment. Her inner child would not speak to her adult self; loving-kindness and understanding words were not enough. Before giving up hope of being able to heal this relationship during the visualization, Michael encouraged Joan to get on her knees, at the level of the little girl. Almost immediately the little girl looked at Joan and began to communicate in a playful way. Being on the same level opened the little girl's joys and fears. A profound sharing and trust was established during this visualization. They held hands, and Joan promised never to abandon her again; she vowed to be her friend and never leave her.

While Michael held the points underneath the base of her skull (GB 20), Joan visualized herself playing with her inner child. As he held her Third Eye, the playfulness turned into a dance, and the walls of the room where she was abused fell away like playing cards. They were left in a gigantic field of yellow sunflowers. The little girl danced joyfully, wearing the same red dancing shoes Joan wore at the party.

Acupressure's safe touch can facilitate trust, increase awareness, and support self-healing. Acupressure points are the gateways to the body's healing energy, which governs self-awareness. But without clear boundaries and intentions, there is always the potential for distrust and additional hurt.

Acupressurists and other bodyworkers, who specialize in emotional balancing, learn ways to handle difficult situations when they are working with survivors of sexual abuse. Emotive therapeutic experiences can occur when the person receiving acupressure breathes deeply as points are held.

Everyone releases and processes their emotions individually and heals at different rates. Since the touch of acupressure has the potential to unleash overpowering feelings, we recommend that you see a psychotherapist to support and deepen your emotional healing process with affirmations and self-acupressure.★

Unconditional love is the embracing of all experience and the bringing of varying intensities to the level of the heart. At the heart level, unconditional love, which is an alive, vibrant state of awareness, replaces the intensities of mood; uncontrolled emotion lifts the energy of these states into a finer, more radiant quality.

— Richard Moss, MD
The I That Is We

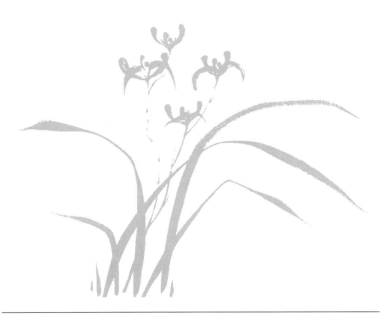

★For more information on emotional and sexual healing for couples, see Michael Reed Gach, PhD, *Acupressure for Lovers* (New York: Bantam Books, 1997).

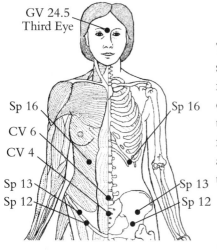

GV 24.5
Third Eye

Sp 16   Sp 16

CV 6

CV 4

Sp 13   Sp 13

Sp 12   Sp 12

MINIROUTINE FOR SEXUAL ABUSE

The following healing visualization is for sexual abuse and incest survivors. (See also Chapter 15.) The acupressure points, healing imagery, and psychological issues it addresses are based on vital energy centers, known as *chakras* in Eastern perspectives of holistic health. We recommend that you work with a psychotherapist for support. Remember to go through the following steps slowly and gently. Practice this or the next acupressure routine several times a week.

Begin in a comfortable position on your back.

Step 1

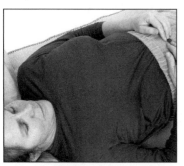

Hold CV 6: This point is located two finger-widths directly below your belly button. Place all your fingertips directly between your navel and pubic bone as you gradually press in one inch deep. Maintain firm pressure while you breathe deeply with your eyes closed. Imagine yourself in your mother's womb, feeling protected, glowing, and supported. Let your body relax by sinking into the earth.

Step 2

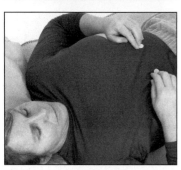

Hold Sp 16: Curve your fingers to press Sp 16 (on the base of your ribcage, in line with the nipples). Gently press upward into the slight indentations for two minutes, and breathe as deeply as you want to heal. Explore how your sexual abuse is related to other issues, such as feeling like you are not being seen or heard.

Step 3

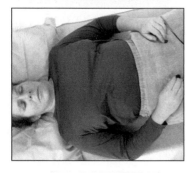

Hold Sp 12 & Sp 13: Using all of your fingertips, press on the ropy ligament in the center of the leg crease at the top of each thigh for one minute. Feel for a strong pulsation from the large artery that runs through these points. Breathe deeply into the core of your hurt, letting whatever pain you feel come out by making a sound; your body no longer needs to store this pain.

Step 4

Hold CV 4 & CV 6: Place the fingertips of one hand just above the center of your pubic bone on CV 4 and the fingers of your other hand between your belly button and pubic bone on CV 6. Close your eyes, and breathe deeply into your abdomen for one minute as you explore how you trust your intuition to support you and keep you safe. As your body relaxes, let yourself go, sinking into and becoming one with the earth. As you continue breathing deeply into your abdomen, trust your newly empowered sense of self.

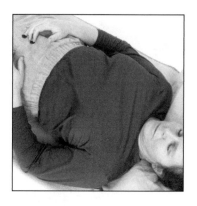

SELF-CARE ROUTINE FOR SEXUAL ABUSE

For safety and for emotional support and guidance, we suggest that you have a trustworthy friend or therapist present while you do the following self-care routine, which will revitalize your creativity and sexuality and heal your emotions.

Begin in a sitting position on a mat or carpeted floor.

Step 1

Acupressure Skull Massage: Massage your skull from the forehead to the base of the skull. Take long, slow, deep breaths as you also massage the sides of your skull thoroughly. Inhale deeply, and hold your breath for three seconds to assimilate the oxygen. Control the flow of air by exhaling slowly through your nose to enhance your experience. Continue long, deep breathing in this manner while you give yourself a good skull massage for three minutes.

We also learn to suffer just to punish whoever abused us . . .

Forgive others, and you will see miracles start to happen in your life.

— Don Miguel Ruiz
The Mastery of Love

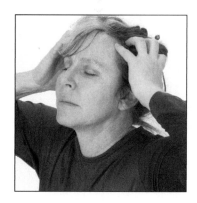

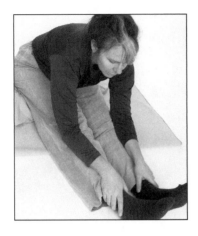

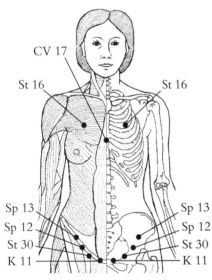

CV 17

St 16   St 16

Sp 13   Sp 13
Sp 12   Sp 12
St 30   St 30
K 11   K 11

Step 2

Leg Stretches: Sit with your legs outstretched in front of you. Extend your hands toward your ankles or feet, and reach forward. Do not strain; stretch as far as you comfortably can. Gently bring your chin toward your knees. Hold for thirty seconds, and relax. Repeat three more times. Focus on deep breathing, inhaling up and exhaling down into the stretch for one minute.

Turn over onto your stomach, lying facedown with your hands comfortably by your sides.

Step 3

Press Sp 12 & Sp 13: Place your fists in your groin over Sp 12 and Sp 13 (where the top of your thigh meets the trunk of your body). Place your forehead on the ground, with your chin tucked into your throat. Inhale deeply, and raise your legs straight up without bending your knees, allowing your body weight to apply pressure to these groin points. Breathe deeply as you focus on this area of your body for one minute to release sexual energy blockages.

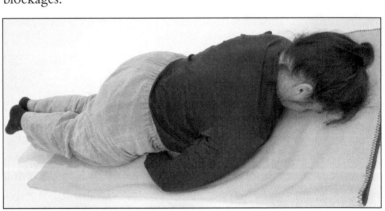

Now roll over onto your back.

Step 4

Hold St 16: Hold this point (located on the chest, below the collarbone, in line with the nipple, just above the breast tissue) for one minute. This is a key nurturing point for developing self-love. Breathe deeply into your belly and then into your chest as you explore your feelings.

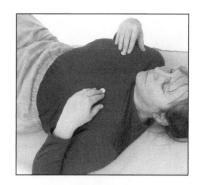

Step 5

Press CV 17 with St 30 & K 11: Place your right hand on CV 17 (at the center of the breastbone) and your left hand on St 30 and K 11 (at the top of the pubic bone). Breathe deeply as you focus on circulating energy throughout your body for a couple of minutes.

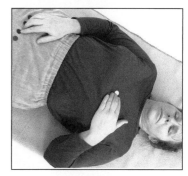

Step 6

Self-Hug: Place the fingertips of each hand into the center of the opposite armpit in a self-hug position and hold for two minutes. This stimulates the H 1 point, cultivating emotional support and spiritual love. Breathe deeply, affirming your ability to love and be sexual. Feel the warmth of your hands surrounding, supporting, and strengthening your heart.

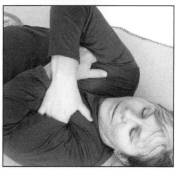

Step 7

Deep Relaxation: To reap the full benefits, rest for five to ten minutes with your hands on your belly, as you breathe deeply.

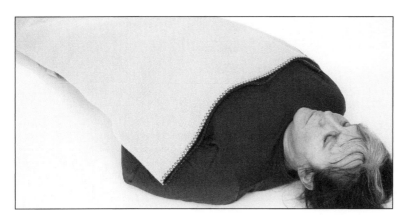

19

STRESS & THE EMOTIONS

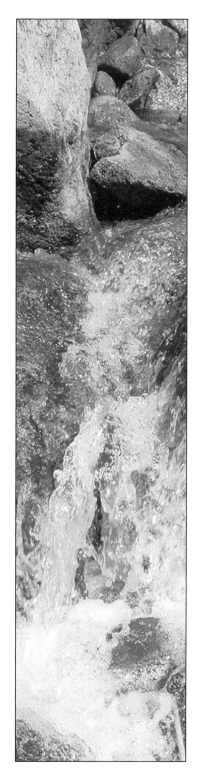

Everybody suffers from stress from time to time, given the tremendous challenges, options, and responsibilities in our busy lives. Your stress may be the result of a long day at work, rush hour traffic, tension with your boss, or a relationship issue. But stress can be exhausting and drain your vital energy, making coping with daily activities difficult.

Stress exacerbates emotional problems and can be the underlying cause of many emotional disorders. If stress is what triggers your emotional imbalances, you may find this chapter pivotal. For instance, if you notice that stress increases your anxiety or worsens the severity of your panic attacks, you could benefit from the point routines in this chapter, as well as those in Chapter 7. In this chapter, you may find some overlap with others in the use of points and techniques, since points benefit multiple problems and stress relates to so many issues.

Stress depresses respiration and causes shallow breathing, which can lead to irritability, frustration, and fatigue. Many people turn to unhealthy habits like smoking, overeating, and excessive drinking to "counteract" stress fallout. Instead, you can use acupressure to transform these hindrances into opportunities for growth. In this chapter you will find hands-on routines to alleviate everyday tensions.

Jenny, a thirty-eight-year-old woman, wrote us, asking how acupressure could relieve her stress and tension. She complained of minor depression, anxiety, occasional insomnia, and headaches. Many of her problems were caused by stress. She had difficulty coping at work and dealing with her marital issues. Her tension, worry, and anxiety made her troubles seem insurmountable.

Affirmations to Counteract Stress

- *I am breathing deeply, as I let go of stress.*

- *With each exhale, I release and relax.*

- *I choose to live in a harmonious way.*

- *Nothing can disturb my inner peace.*

- *I can handle whatever comes to me.*

- *I no longer need to hold on to stress; stress no longer serves me.*

Overwhelming feelings drove her to eat compulsively. Jenny's life was in such a rut that she felt helpless and incapacitated.

We suggested she practice the self-care routine in this chapter for twenty minutes each morning and each evening for three weeks. She did so and wrote the following about the changes and feelings she experienced as a result:

"Only weeks ago overwhelming anxiety attacks created great hardships for me. I now feel the 'mud' around my heart lifting; my body seems to be filtering out toxins held for years. Giving myself acupressure not only helped me realize many of the causes of my stress, such as holding my breath at work, but also has enabled me to handle stressful situations with greater ease. Instead of doubting myself and holding back, I feel more empowered to express what is going on with me. When I notice my body tensing, I hold a few key points and almost immediately experience a greater sense of serenity—at home, while stuck in traffic, in the midst of a meeting with my boss or at a social event. I've found acupressure a great blessing for my busy professional and personal life."

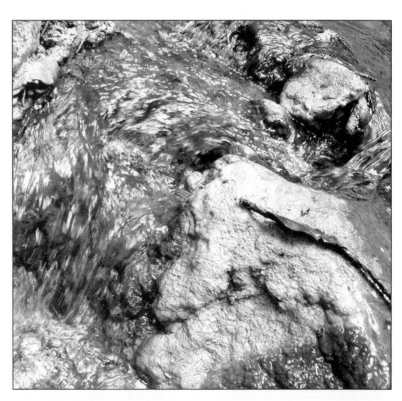

QUICK TIPS FOR STRESS

Once you practice these easy hands-on techniques and become familiar with them, teach them to your children or friends to enable them to manage stress and frustration, too.

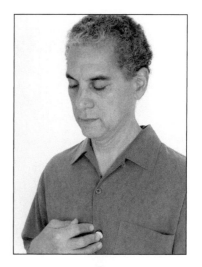

Sea of Tranquility (CV 17): Hold this point (in the indentations in the center of your breastbone) when you feel frustrated, irritated, or tense. Holding this emotional balancing point releases uptightness in the chest and enables deep breathing. Use your fingertips to hold CV 17 for three minutes, as you breathe slowly and deeply for an instant calming effect whenever you feel agitated or under stress.

You can repeat this simple but effective technique many times throughout the day when you want to calm yourself. Try it the next time you feel frustrated, irritated, nervous, or anxious. The more you practice this technique, the more the Sea of Tranquility point will open for achieving inner peace and improve the quality of your life.

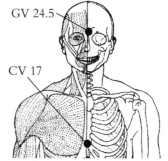

Third Eye Point (GV 24.5): Use this point to transform negative emotions during stressful times. Close your eyes, and gently place your middle fingertip between your eyebrows on GV 24.5 (in the slight indentation just above the bridge of your nose). To collect your thoughts and rejuvenate yourself, breathe slowly and deeply for three minutes as you focus your attention on the gentle touch of this point. This touch meditation can shift your state of mind and revitalize you in just three minutes.

Co-Counseling

Joining a co-counseling group is a safe, inexpensive way to process emotional distress, resentment, and other unfinished feelings. These groups teach supportive active listening and can be an effective way to release your emotions. See Appendix D for more information.

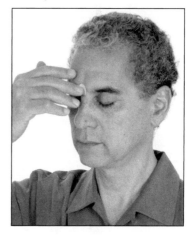

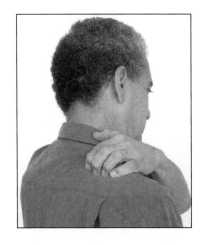

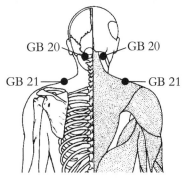

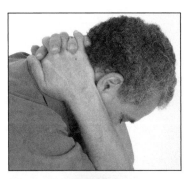

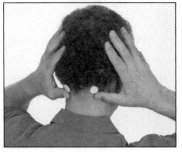

SELF-CARE ROUTINE FOR STRESS

This acupressure routine releases shoulder and neck tension and can transform stress into a sense of well-being. Although this routine is shown sitting, you can also practice these techniques lying down.

Step 1

Shoulder Grasp: Curve your fingers, of both hands, and place them on the tops of your shoulder muscles (GB 21), close to the base of your neck. Gradually apply firm pressure directly on to your shoulder tension. Simply let the weight of your arms relax forward, keeping your fingers curved like a hook. Sink deeply into the muscles as they soften and relax. Hold for one minute as you take slow, deep breaths. Then let your hands relax in your lap. Gently shrug your shoulders up and down several times to encourage them to relax further.

Variation: You can also practice the Shoulder Grasp using one hand at a time. Place your right fingertips on your left shoulder, grasp and hold for a minute, then switch to press the other side.

Step 2

Neck Press: Interlace your fingers behind your neck, and let your head hang forward, with your elbows close together, pointing down toward your lap. Inhale deeply, raising your head as you stretch your elbows out to the sides; let your head tilt back. Exhale as your head relaxes forward and your elbows come close together in front of you. Repeat this exercise for two minutes; then let your hands float back into your lap. Keeping your eyes closed, take another minute to let yourself relax deeply.

Step 3

Press GB 20: Close your eyes, and place your thumbs on GB 20 (underneath the base of your skull in the indentations that lie about three inches apart). Apply firm pressure for one minute.

Step 4

Press St 6: Place your fingertips on the jaw muscles to firmly press St 6. You should feel a muscle pop out when you clench your molars together. Hold these points firmly on the jaw muscle with your teeth slightly apart, breathing deeply, for one minute. End with thirty seconds of light pressure as you continue breathing deeply.

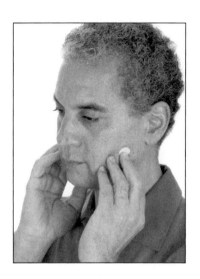

Step 5

Touch GV 24.5 with CV 17: Gently place your right middle fingertip on GV 24.5 (in between your eyebrows, in the indentation where the bridge of your nose meets your forehead). Position the fingertips of your left hand on CV 17 (in the indentation of your breastbone at the level of your heart). Close your eyes as you hold these points, and breathe deeply for at least one minute.

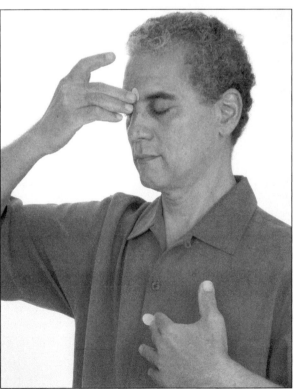

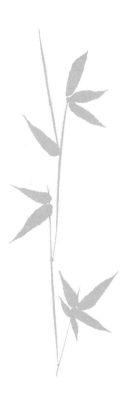

Step 6

Deeply Relax: Relax for five to ten minutes with your eyes closed, letting the energy circulate throughout your body, to gain the full benefits.

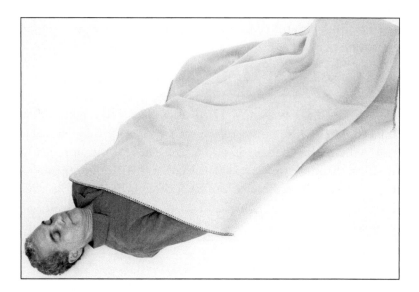

20

TRAUMA & POST-TRAUMATIC STRESS DISORDER

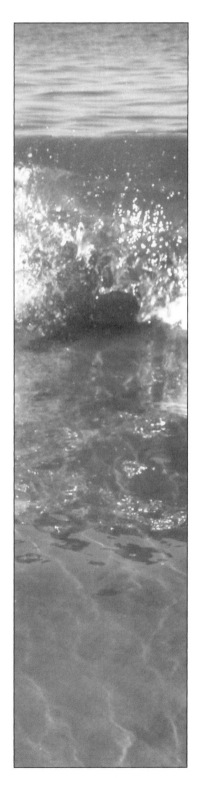

When traumatic experiences are unresolved, tension accumulates, and repressed memories can develop into physical symptoms. Whether the nature of the trauma is predominantly emotional or physical, your body holds in its musculature a range of emotions from mild to severe. A mild emotional trauma can be caused by your parents yelling at you as a child or a teacher reprimanding you in class. A divorce or a time when your boss ridiculed you can also be emotionally traumatic. A more severe case of emotional trauma is the sudden loss of a parent or long-term and constant psychological abuse by a parent or spouse. For instance, a father who tells his daughter that she is "ugly, stupid, and unwanted" and "I wish you were dead" is heaping emotional and verbal abuse on her. There are many causes of physical trauma: a serious car accident; being mugged, kidnapped, robbed, or raped; or the terrors of war.

Both emotionally and physically traumatic experiences can cause fear, shock, and emotional numbness (see Chapter 11). If you are hurt, frightened, or in physical pain, your body may naturally dissociate from your feelings. The body physically responds by contracting the muscles as a protective mechanism since the experience is too painful to assimilate in the moment. Unless the muscles are released, the feelings remain inaccessible. They are stored in your memories, and your memories are stored in the cells of your body, to be dealt with later. If these emotions are not processed, numerous ailments and problems may result. The severity of the trauma equals the severity of the emotional or physical symptoms. But, the sooner acupressure treatments are

Affirmations to Counteract Trauma & PTSD

- *I am safe and secure.*

- *I am grateful to be alive.*

- *I trust my body to heal itself.*

- *I let go of the past and am renewed.*

- *I have faith that I am being taken care of.*

- *I am living in the present moment now and release my past traumas.*

started, followed by deep relaxation, the quicker you will be able to heal and recover from the trauma, thus preventing post-traumatic stress disorder. When your acupressure points are held and you are supported to relax and breathe deeply, your feelings can resurface, allowing the healing process to begin.

Use visualization along with self-acupressure to go deeper in your healing, both on your own and with a psychotherapist who incorporates mind-body techniques. You cannot heal an emotional wound without exploring the painful memories and negative feelings connected to it. Healing from a trauma is especially powerful when the acupressure points are simply held. A profound experience often occurs as the energy flowing from one point to another reawakens traumatic memories stored within the body.

Making sounds and using other forms of expression, such as journaling or artwork, are effective for releasing emotional pain. Be sure to continue to come back to your body awareness as you explore past memories. In this process, your healing is attained by breathing slowly, evenly, and deeply. If your emotions become overwhelming or you find yourself getting dizzy or feel out of control, hold CV 17 and GV 26, as described in this chapter. For severe trauma, an acupressurist and somatic psychotherapist who works with the breath and the mind-body connection is highly recommended to engage with this level of emotional healing.

Carry was kidnapped and held at knifepoint for three days. She was raped, beaten, and terrorized. She had three broken ribs, bruises, and a broken jaw. She was frightened, numb, and unable to speak or make eye contact with anyone. Carry's sister, an acupressure student of Beth's, made an emergency call to her from the emergency ward at the hospital. Carry's sister knew the beneficial applications of acupressure in releasing emotional trauma and wanted Carry to have an appointment immediately.

Carry received acupressure therapy every day for one week, in conjunction with medical and psychological treatment, while she was hospitalized. She learned deep breathing skills, received hand and foot massages, used affirmations, and focused on deep relaxation. She practiced the simple miniroutines in this chapter twice a day. She slept soundly at night without taking sleep medication by using a gentle self-acupressure technique, with her palms over her heart holding the point on the center of her breastbone (CV 17). It eased her fear and anxiety. Beth encouraged her to cry and moan instead of avoiding her pain.

Even though Carry's body had bruises and broken bones, she used gentle acupressure instead of medications for pain relief. After just ten days she recovered her strength and spirit. Acupressure along with psychotherapy discharged the trauma from being kidnapped and relaxed her deeply enough that she could deal with the horrible ordeal and heal her emotional wounds. The fast recovery was a blessing to her children and family.

The quick results from acupressure and deep breathing contributed greatly to Carry's speedy recovery. Storing the memories in her body could have resulted in muscle contractions and nervous disorders, but acupressure kept the energy moving to facilitate her healing process. Continuing to use self-acupressure on a regular basis for maintenance helped her to prevent post-traumatic stress.

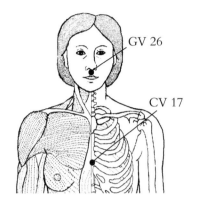

Both trauma and post-traumatic stress retain the experiences in the musculature, but post-traumatic stress disorder is more extreme and jolting to the nervous system. An emotional trauma may not necessarily involve shocking the system. The trauma may involve emotional pain and fear but not terror and horror, which strangles the nervous system and is often the cause of post-traumatic stress. For example, the process of divorce or being ridiculed by your boss can be emotionally traumatic but is less likely to produce post-traumatic stress symptoms.

Post-Traumatic Stress Disorder (PTSD)

Post-traumatic stress is a disorder resulting from shock or trauma that causes multiple symptoms, including any combination of flashbacks, nightmares, anxiety, depression, anger, negativity, suspiciousness, panic, and chronic physical pain. Survivors of war and victims of abuse often suffer from severe post-traumatic stress. Many psychological problems can be related to unexpressed, unhealed trauma.

The body's neuromuscular system registers traumatic and painful memories in the form of physical stress. This can disrupt the body's internal balance, affecting its functions adversely and

Trauma arises because the pain involved in the event has not been faced and experienced.... Ironically, our thoughts become the shield from our feelings. Even though we think about the event, we still do not integrate the feelings, which continue to haunt us.

— John Ruskan
Emotional Clearing

An essential part of healing from traumatic experiences is to express and share your feelings. When you were young, you could not do this. You suppressed those feelings but you have not gotten rid of them.

— Ellen Bass and Laura Davis
The Courage to Heal

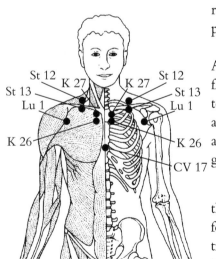

St 12
K 27   K 27   St 12
St 13   St 13
Lu 1   Lu 1
K 26   K 26
CV 17

causing multiple health problems. Like a time capsule, PTSD can be triggered years after the traumatic incident by situations that resemble it.

Post-traumatic stress can be relieved over time using acupressure, yoga, deep breathing techniques, and the support of a good counselor or psychotherapist. When the points open, healing energy flows, creating an involuntary release; the body may shake, tremble, yawn, sigh, or cry. Related images and memories that surface are often a reexperience of the original trauma. Once memories and feelings are released and processed through these therapeutic activities, post-traumatic symptoms begin to fade.

Gordon, a Vietnam veteran with PTSD, had anxiety, flashbacks, cold sweats, and severe nightmares. These symptoms had tremendous impact on his relationships. He was a loner; no one understood the extent of his ongoing problems. His symptoms prevented him from forming long-term intimate relationships. His nightmares and lack of sleep left him feeling exhausted and irritable for days. Depression increased his negative thinking and caused him to socially isolate himself. He had difficulty concentrating or finishing tasks, especially at work. At times his body would break out in hives and cause intense itching all over. Since returning from war, Gordon also suffered from terrible digestive problems and felt miserable for days at a time.

Gordon had a mixed reaction to his first acupressure session. Although he enjoyed the deep relaxation, the vividness of his flashbacks frightened him. But psychotherapy encouraged him to continue to work on healing his PTSD. He also learned yoga and practiced self-acupressure at home. Gordon described his acupressure and psychotherapy as "a way of dumping the garbage" he had seen in Vietnam, watching his friends get killed.

Psychotherapists have found vivid memories to be useful in the emotional healing process of patients with PTSD.★ We have found that acupressure increases a client's ability to visualize past traumatic events. Holding the points steady for several minutes increases circulation and levels of endorphins, neurochemicals that naturally release pain. As the points are held, body awareness and the ability to visualize past experiences can fully awaken.

★Mardi Horowitz, MD, *American Journal of Psychiatry,* (September 1985).

To release the muscular armor resulting from Gordon's trauma, he massaged and then held the following acupressure points for two minutes each:

GB 21 (On the top of the shoulders, directly below the earlobes): Feeling for the tightest portion of the shoulder muscle and applying firm pressure, Gordon breathed slowly and deeply to release his tension.

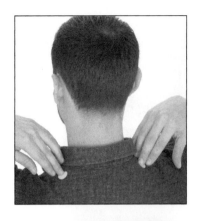

SI 10 (In the upper back, where the arms and shoulder blades meet, two inches up from the back of the armpit crease): Gordon crossed his arms in front of himself and reached around, as if hugging his body, to hook his fingers into SI 10.

B 10 (In the upper neck on the tightest spot, one thumb-width out from the center of the spine): Gordon curved his fingers to hook into the tightest part of the upper neck muscles, which released his traumatic stress.

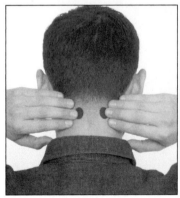

Gordon discovered that holding points on his chest (K 26, K 27, St 12, St 13, and Lu 1) below the collarbone made him feel calmer and less agitated. Holding CV 17, on the center of his breastbone, increased his capacity to breathe deeply. This reduced his anxiety and depression, and calmed his mind. He also learned the most effective ways to hold these points.

Gordon used acupressure for self-treatment several times daily for three- to five-minute intervals. Within three months he felt he was finally able to function like a normal human being again, without 90 percent of his mental disorientation and other post-traumatic stress symptoms.

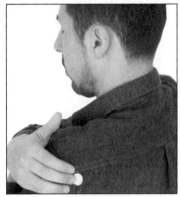

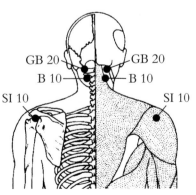

> *While trauma can be hell on earth, trauma resolved is a gift of the gods—a heroic journey that belongs to each of us.*
>
> — Peter A. Levine
> *Waking the Tiger*

LIFESTYLE CONSIDERATIONS

Traditional Chinese medicine teaches the following lifestyle changes for balancing emotional distress:

Eat Plenty of Green Vegetables: This means both lightly steamed and raw. The minerals, vitamins, chlorophyll, and life energy contained in green vegetables can stabilize your emotions.

Consciously Reduce Oil in Your Diet: Excessive oil taxes the liver and hinders emotional balance. Avoid potato chips, French fries, fried chicken, and other fried foods.

Avoid Eating Sugar: This will stabilize your system and emotions.

Stretch Throughout the Day: This will enhance circulation, keep your muscles toned, and increase your vitality.

QUICK TIPS FOR
TRAUMA & PTSD

If you don't have enough time to practice all of the following activities, practicing only one or two of them can be beneficial.

Foot Massage: Acupressure points located in the foot nourish and relax the whole body. Massage your feet for two minutes each while breathing deeply, for post-trauma, postsurgery, and the general reduction of pain.

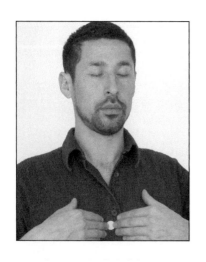

Press CV 17: If fearful memories surface and you feel overwhelmed or unsafe, anxiety and panic can paralyze your breathing or cause you to hyperventilate. If this occurs, press Sea of Tranquility (CV 17, located on the breastbone, four fingerwidths above its base, at the level of the heart). Press into the indentations with your fingers while breathing deeply, through your nose if possible. Encourage yourself to relax as you continue to focus on breathing slowly and deeply for two minutes. Breathing slowly through your nose counteracts hyperventilation. Holding this emotional balancing point can open your chest, increase respiration, and stabilize a panic or anxiety attack.

Rub St 36: Place your right fist on the outside of your right leg and your left fist on the outside of your left leg. Briskly rub up and down beside the shinbone for one minute as you breathe deeply into your belly. Focus on exhaling completely to discharge any emotional residue. St 36 is effective for dizziness, anxiety, palpitations, and the dissociation commonly reported after trauma.

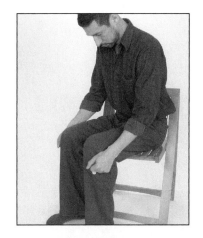

Hold P 8: Press the point in the middle of your palm with the opposite fingertips or thumb. This is a strong emotional balancing point for harmonizing the mind and spirit after trauma. Switch and press your other side.

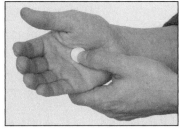

Stretch: Take five to ten minutes to gently stretch sore, tense areas of your body. Stretching is important, since dealing with traumatic memories can cause painful muscle contractions and stiffness. Stretching your muscles increases circulation and tones the body; physical flexibility supports both spiritual and emotional resilience.

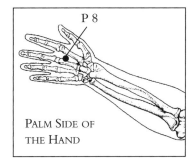

P 8

PALM SIDE OF THE HAND

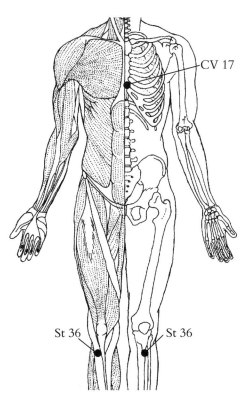

CV 17

St 36   St 36

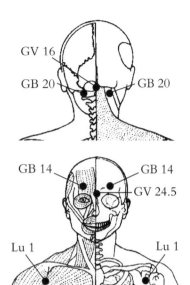

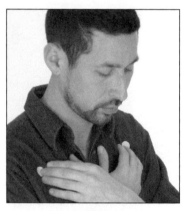

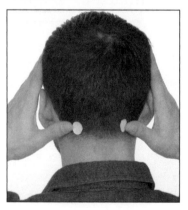

SPECIAL POINTS FOR RELIEVING TRAUMA & POST-TRAUMATIC STRESS

If you suffer from PTSD, anxiety, or panic attacks, follow a few simple rules during your first few weeks of self-acupressure. Ask a trusted friend or family member to stay by your side and limit the amount of time you hold these points to one minute each. If you are having violent images or suicidal thoughts (or taking antidepressants), do not use these points alone without your support person. Concentrate on breathing slowly, fully, and deeply. At the same time hold one or more of the following acupressure points for calming yourself:

Letting Go (Lu 1)

Location: On the outer part of the chest, four finger-widths up from the armpit crease and one finger-width inward.

Instructions: Cross your arms over the center of your chest, and place your fingertips firmly on both sides of your outer chest for two minutes. As you hold these emotional healing points, breathe deeply.

Benefits: Relieves difficult breathing, trauma, stress, fatigue, confusion, emotional repression, choking, and asthma.

Gates of Consciousness (GB 20)

Location: Just below the base of the skull, in the hollow between the two large neck muscles, three inches apart.

Instructions: Use your thumbs to press underneath the base of your skull into the indentations on both sides. Slowly tilt your head back with your eyes closed. Imagine that this mental balancing point is relieving your panic and anxiety as you gently press up underneath your skull for one to two minutes and take slow, deep breaths.

Benefits: Relieves headaches, neck stiffness and pain, trauma, shock, hypertension, and irritability.

Wind Mansion (GV 16)

Location: At the base of the skull, in the large center hollow.

Instructions: Place your middle fingers on the points, and close your eyes. Slowly tilt your head back, and breathe deeply as you press firmly into this hollow area for one minute.

Benefits: Relieves headaches, pain, insomnia, shock, trauma, stiff neck, head congestion, and mental stress.

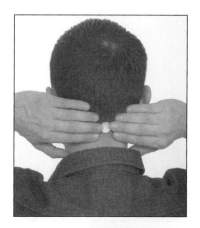

Third Eye (GV 24.5)

Location: Between the eyebrows, in the indentation where the bridge of the nose joins the forehead.

Instructions: Sitting with your spine straight, eyes closed, and chin tilted down slightly, bring your palms together, and use your middle and index fingertips to lightly touch the Third Eye point. Take long, slow, deep breaths for one minute as you visualize yourself in a place that makes you feel calm, restful, and safe— where you can trust yourself to follow whatever steps you need to heal your past traumas.

Benefits: Relieves pain, headaches, dizziness, emotional instability, irritability, and confusion. Balances the pituitary gland, the master endocrine gland that secretes hormones and neurochemicals to relieve anxiety.

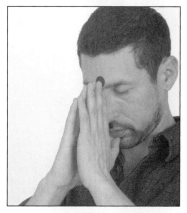

Clear Mind (GB 14)

Location: One finger-width above the eyebrows, in line with the center of the iris.

Instructions: Place your thumb on one side and your third finger on the other to gently stimulate GB 14 on both sides. Use the lightest touch possible on these emotional balancing points.

Benefits: Relieves pain, shock, and trauma and clears the mind.

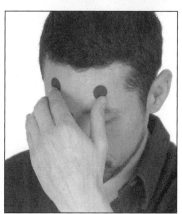

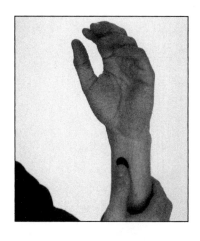

Inner Gate (P 6)

Location: Three finger-widths up from the center of the inner wrist crease.

Instructions: Place your right thumb on the point. Position your fingertips on the outside directly behind your thumb, and firmly grasp for one minute as you breathe deeply. Then switch wrists and hold for another minute.

Benefits: Relieves nervousness, shock, trauma, nausea, insomnia, palpitations, and wrist pain; calms emotional upset and balances your inner world.

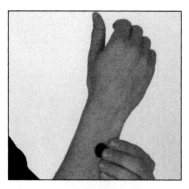

Outer Gate (TW 5)

Location: Three finger-widths above the outer wrist crease, between the two forearm bones.

Instructions: Position your fingertips on the point. Firmly grasp TW 5 with P 6 for one minute as you breathe deeply, then switch wrists and hold for another minute.

Benefits: Relieves pain in the shoulder and wrist; boosts the immune system and harmonizes social relationships.

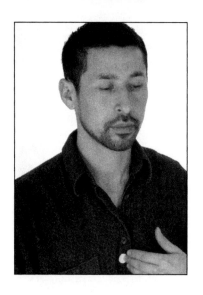

Sea of Tranquility (CV 17)

Location: On the center of your breastbone, four finger-widths up from the base of the sternum.

Instructions: Use your fingertips to hold the point. As you do so, use your mind to concentrate on taking slow, deep breaths into your heart for three minutes.

Benefits: This emotional balancing point opens the chest for deep breathing, activates the thymus gland, and is especially good for counteracting anxiety.

Balanced Love (P 9)

Location: At the base of the middle fingernail.

Instructions: Hold this point firmly, and take long, slow, deep breaths for three minutes.

Benefits: Can instantly calm a panic attack and comfort your emotions.

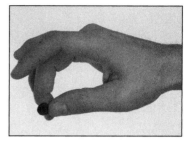

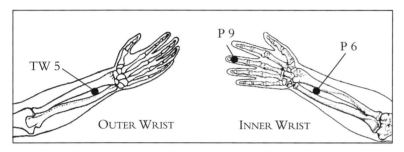

TW 5

P 9

P 6

OUTER WRIST   INNER WRIST

Center of the Person (GV 26)

Location: Two-thirds of the way up from the upper lip to the nose.

Instructions: Use your index or middle fingertip to press firmly on GV 26, angling the pressure into your upper gum. Breathe deeply as you hold the point for two minutes.

Benefits: Reduces emotional shock, revives consciousness, calms the spirit, and improves memory and concentration. Also relieves dizziness, nosebleeds, muscle cramps, and pain.

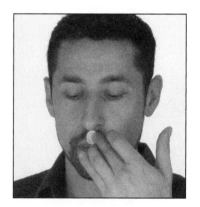

Sea of Energy (CV 6)

Location: Three finger-widths below the navel.

Instructions: Place all of your fingertips on the point. Gradually press in one inch deep. Maintain this firm pressure while breathing deeply into your belly with your eyes closed.

Benefits: Relieves trauma, extreme fatigue, dizziness, general weakness, and confusion. With deep abdominal breathing, fosters security and emotional stability.

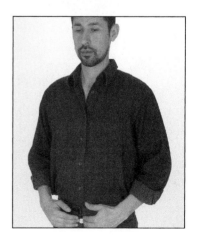

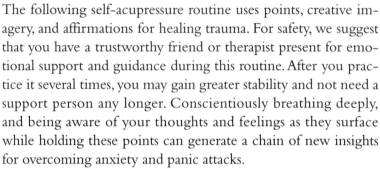

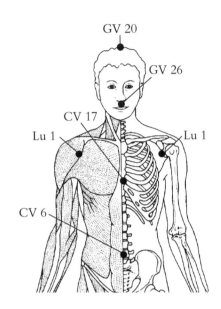

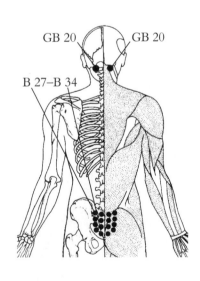

SELF-CARE ROUTINE FOR
TRAUMA & PTSD

The following self-acupressure routine uses points, creative imagery, and affirmations for healing trauma. For safety, we suggest that you have a trustworthy friend or therapist present for emotional support and guidance during this routine. After you practice it several times, you may gain greater stability and not need a support person any longer. Conscientiously breathing deeply, and being aware of your thoughts and feelings as they surface while holding these points can generate a chain of new insights for overcoming anxiety and panic attacks.

This routine should not be used without professional support, if you are taking antidepressant drugs, feel out of control, or have flashbacks that previously caused hospitalization, additional trauma, or emotional instability. Unresolved emotionally traumatic experiences can cause you to dissociate from your body. This can make your breathing shallow and lead to obsessive worry, self-doubt, or overwhelming feelings. If you notice this, compassionately remind yourself to deepen and slow down your breath; be more attentive to your body.

If you begin to feel anxious, confused, or out of control, palm the CV 17 point over the center of your breastbone with both hands. You can also hold one hand on CV 17 and the other hand on your lower belly to press CV 6; breathe slowly and deeply until you feel stable. The purpose of using deep breathing is to keep your body's vital energy circulating and enhance your awareness; increased awareness is vital for emotional healing.

Roll a towel up firmly, then place it between your shoulder blades as you lie down on your back comfortably.

Step 1

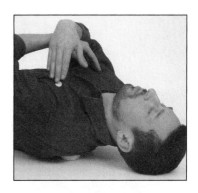

Press Lu 1: Cross your wrists in front of the center of your chest, and place your fingertips on the Letting Go point (Lu 1, on the upper, outer part of the chest). Rub your chest muscles to feel for the tightest spot, and place your middle fingertips on the "knot." Adjust the towel between your shoulder blades to apply a firm but comfortable pressure in your upper back. Firmly hold these Letting Go points as you concentrate on breathing deeply for one to three minutes.

Step 2

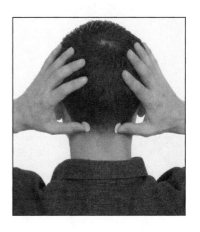

Press GB 20: Place your thumbs underneath the base of your skull, in the indentations that lie three inches apart. Slowly tilt your head as you gradually press up and under the skull with your eyes closed. Take long, slow, deep breaths as you direct the pressure firmly upward and inward to connect with the Gates of Consciousness (GB 20). Continue to breathe deeply as you recall the time when you were traumatized. View your memories like a movie. Take a couple of minutes to review what happened. Use this imagery to go deeper in your healing, both with yourself and later with a psychotherapist. Let yourself relax and breathe deeply as you hold GB 20 for one to three minutes or until you feel a regular, even pulse on both sides. Continue to breathe into your feelings as you slowly release the pressure.

Step 3

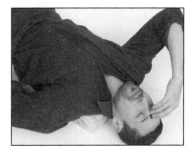

Hold Sacral Points B 27 to B 34 with Balancing Points: Place one hand palm up, under the base of the spine, so the weight of your body presses points B 27 through B 34. Use your other hand to hold the following balancing points for one minute each, while breathing slowly and deeply:

- **GV 20:** Place all your fingertips in the center of the top of your head, in the dip at the crown.

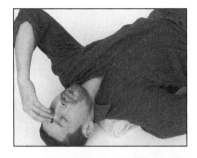

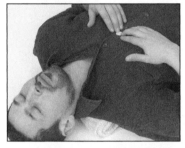

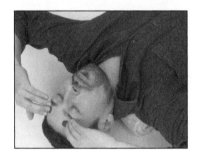

- **GV 24.5:** Place your middle fingertip lightly in between your eyebrows on GV 24.5 (in the indentation where the bridge of your nose meets the ridge of your forehead). Focus your attention on that spot with your eyes closed. Breathe deeply for two minutes as you hold this nervous system balancing point.

- **CV 17:** Place all your fingertips on the center of your breastbone at heart level, fitting them into each of the indentations. Close your eyes, and breathe deeply. Concentrate on making each breath grow longer and deeper than the last one. Breathe out any tension… Feel your mind clear with each breath; notice the resistance, worries, and judgments your mind creates… With each exhalation, let go of these attitudes… Remember to breathe deeply—bringing life energy into your body, the essence that can heal you...

Step 4

Forehead Touch: Gently touch GB 14 on both sides (one finger-width up from the eyebrow, directly above the center of your eyeball). Holding this emotional balancing point reprograms your mental patterns, calms your mind from painful memories, and clears away the fear and shock of trauma.

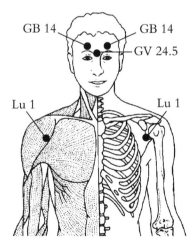

Step 5

Take a Nap: Cover yourself with a blanket, and lie down on your back. Close your eyes, bring your hands onto your belly, and make yourself comfortable to deeply relax for at least five to ten minutes. When you are ready to return, bend and hug your knees while you rock back and forth on your spine for a minute. Then roll up to a comfortable sitting position.

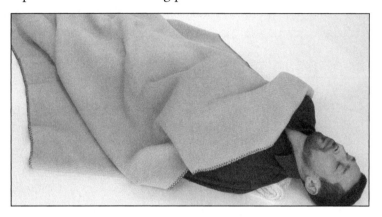

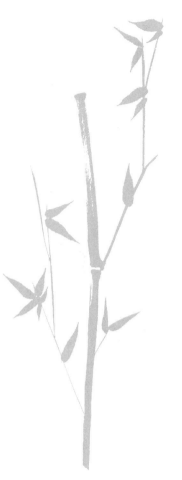

Step 6

Foot Massage: Squeeze all parts of your feet, covering the arches, balls of the feet, heels, and finally toes. Massaging the feet while breathing deeply for two minutes promotes emotional stability.

21

WORRY & SELF-DOUBT

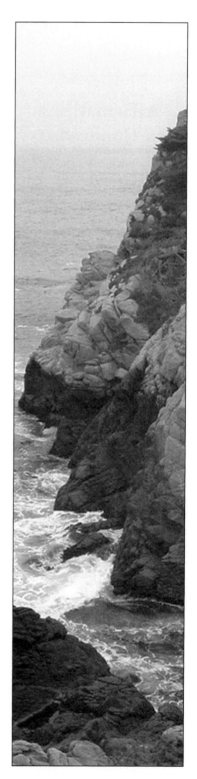

Worry and self-doubt can drain your vital energy and take you away from the present moment, causing discord between your mind and body. Worry entraps energy in your head, causing excessive thinking and headaches; this can be especially overwhelming when an expectation creates more mental barriers and further divides the mind from the body. Physically, worry and self-doubt tax the spleen, pancreas, and other digestive organs, causing problems such as hyperacidity, poor digestion, ulcers, stomachaches, eating disorders, and food cravings. In Chinese medicine, working on the Spleen meridian points balances energy and counteracts the physical and behavioral problems associated with worry and self-doubt.

Exercising daily and using deep breathing along with the self-acupressure routines in this chapter counteract worry and affirm your self-worth. Use your willpower, set your goals, and consistently focus on affirmations and other positive thoughts. Having compassion for yourself is the first step toward having compassion and loving-kindness for others.

Sheila, a longtime client, suffered with self-doubt, worry, headaches, mood swings, and digestive imbalances. Her voice and facial expressions showed excessive concern with having to do everything right. When she began the self-acupressure program, her digestive problems were at their peak; there were only four or five foods she could eat without feeling ulcer pain. She spent many days lying in bed unable to eat or move. She had not determined the source of her digestive disturbances; she only knew her symptoms worsened when she was under the stress of worrisome thoughts.

Affirmations to Counteract Worry & Self-Doubt

- *I trust my perceptions and intuition.*

- *I let go of being perfect.*

- *I love and accept myself as I am.*

- *I am worthy of love.*

- *I have faith in myself.*

Sheila expected herself to be perfect in the workplace, in her marriage, and in her role as a parent. Her compulsive nature made life stressful and competitive. She often rushed into her appointments late, complaining about every aspect of her life. Her pace and tone of voice were always urgent, no matter what the subject matter. The continual chatter in her mind made relaxation difficult.

Worry was a childhood pattern for Sheila; she grew up in a family devoid of emotional intimacy, support, and nurturing. Her mother was particularly negative, was chronically depressed, and did not show affection. Her mother's mood swings and unpredictability were partially responsible for Sheila's insecurities and lack of self-esteem.

Sheila's father was a workaholic; he also suffered from severe arthritic pain. When he was at home, he was often noncommunicative or sleeping. His unresponsiveness, coupled with his wife's emotional unavailability, fostered Sheila's feelings of uncertainty and anxiety. Since she got no attention or feedback at home, her self-esteem suffered, which also made her vulnerable to being taken for granted by others.

During childhood, the following cycle commonly occurs: the child desires to please the parent; if the parent is unapproachable, the child tries even harder. When attempts to please are unsuccessful, worry and obsession can result.

Sheila's childhood experiences contributed to her obsessive behavior. Since she was six years old, she worried about other people's lives, unconsciously hoping this would make people love her and ultimately satisfy her childhood needs for emotional support. Loneliness was not as haunting when she was meeting others' needs. She became a compulsive mother by attempting to be perfect, encouraging her kids to be dependent on her.

Sheila's emotional healing process involved recognizing and accepting her sadness and lack of love as a child. Through awareness she saw how her blocked emotions created physical symptoms. The fear of not being special enough to be loved was the underlying cause of her compulsions and excessive sweetness.

Acupressure provided Sheila with a safe way to focus on her body and emotions. By using points, stretching, deep breathing, and affirmations, she was able to heal the parts of herself that were wounded as a child.

Sheila often felt like crying during her self-acupressure routines. At first this made her feel uneasy about her daily practice, but by paying attention to and experiencing her sadness, she was able to appreciate her feelings more. Crying was vital for releasing her negative self-image and lack of confidence.

The security of acupressure's touch fostered trust, self-love, and increased awareness in Sheila. Instead of relying on drugs with harmful side effects, she preferred self-acupressure. After her physical symptoms resolved completely, she continued her home program on a daily basis to maintain her new emotional stability and strength.

DIETARY CONSIDERATIONS

Gentle foods and herbs can combat hyperacidity, heartburn, and food allergies. Use the following guidelines.

- **Herbs:** Mint, ginger, fennel, and licorice root can counteract hyperacidity. Add two ounces of one or a combination of all these herbs to one quart of boiled water. Let the herb tea steep for fifteen to twenty minutes. Drink a cup of this tea after each meal.

- **Avoid Sugar:** Eat good-quality sweet foods, such as yams, squash, brown rice, cooked or raw carrots, and apples. If a sweetener is necessary, use a small amount of molasses, fruit juice, or stevia (a naturally sweet herb available at health food stores). Avoid too much fruit, fruit juice, and soda.

- **Use Spice:** Eating ginger, cinnamon, garlic, onion, and a small amount of cayenne pepper dries out dampness in your body and encourages digestion during times of stress.

- **Avoid Iced Products:** Eating too much cold food, including iced drinks, inhibits digestion.

- **Decrease Mucus-Forming Foods:** Dairy products, heavy proteins combined with starch, nut butters, gravies, and hydrogenated oils cause sluggishness and can trigger worrisome emotions.

When doubt arises, which it does over and over again, it becomes a signal that it is time to let go, rebalance and find an unconditional allowing of life.

— Richard Moss, MD
The I That Is We

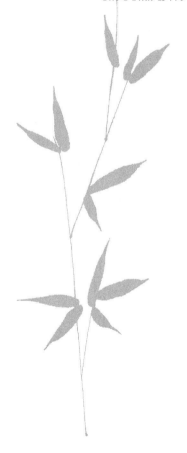

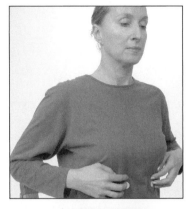

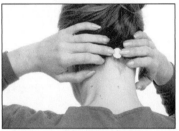

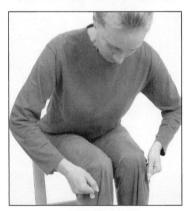

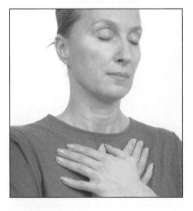

ACUPRESSURE POINTS FOR
WORRY & SELF-DOUBT

- **Sp 16** (below the edge of the ribcage, directly below the nipple line): Holding this key point opens circulation through the waistline, governs appetite and digestion, and balances self-esteem, worry, sadness, grief, codependent patterns, and abandonment. Breathe deeply into your belly for two minutes as you focus your awareness on the movement of healing energy through this area.

- **GV 16** (in the center back of the head, in the large hollow under the base of the skull): Holding this key point clears the mind of obsessive thoughts, and opens the head, neck, and throat. It also relieves insomnia, trauma, shock, hypertension, headaches, neck pain, and dizziness. Hold this point lightly for one to three minutes.

- **St 36** (four finger-widths below the kneecap, toward the outside shinbone): St 36 aids mental confusion, self-doubt, worrisome thoughts, overwhelming emotion, and digestive stress and tension. To stabilize your thoughts and emotions, briskly rub both points with your fists for one minute.

- **CV 17** (on the center of the breastbone four finger-widths up from the base of the sternum): Holding this key point opens the chest and calms and relaxes the entire body, reducing nervousness and anxiety. It also relieves depression, sadness, and melancholy by increasing circulation to the cardiovascular system. Palm this area with one hand over the other to nourish your spirit and clear your mind of worrisome thoughts. CV 17 supports deep emotional and spiritual healing.

MINIROUTINE FOR
WORRY & SELF-DOUBT

This routine takes only five minutes and is most effective to do throughout the day, whenever you catch yourself worrying.

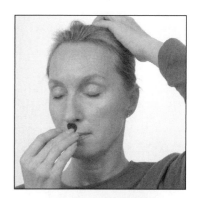

Step 1

Hold GV 20 with GV 26: Place your fingertips on the back of your ears, then glide them up to the top of your head in the center, to lightly touch GV 20. This point lies in an indentation on the skull; it is the soft spot on a baby. Use the middle finger of your other hand to press into the gum between your upper lip and nose (GV 26). Straighten your spine, and take long, slow, deep breaths for one minute to transform your worry.

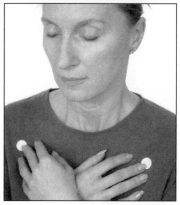

Step 2

Hold Lu 1: Place both hands on opposite Lu 1 points in the upper, outer chest region. Holding Lu 1 aids in letting go. Breathe deeply into these points, breathing out any worrisome thoughts, for two minutes. Make the sound of *ahhh* on the exhalation to further release your stress and tension.

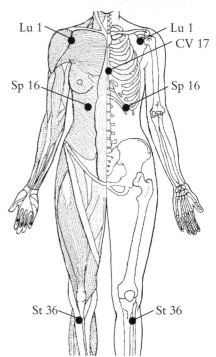

Step 3

Rub St 36: Briskly rub St 36 on both legs with your knuckles, four finger-widths below the kneecap, one finger-width outside of both shinbones, for two minutes. Doing this several times throughout the day can eliminate worry and give you greater energy.

Step 4

Brisk Walk: If you have time, walk briskly, breathing deeply as you swing your arms vigorously for a few minutes. You can do this indoors or outdoors.

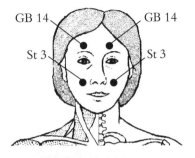

GB 14   GB 14

St 3   St 3

SELF-CARE ROUTINE FOR
WORRY & SELF-DOUBT

Treat yourself with this routine daily, followed by deep relaxation. To begin, lie down comfortably on your back.

Step 1

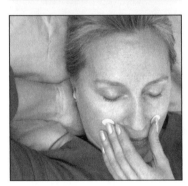

Hold B 10 with GB 14: Place the palm of your right hand over the back of your neck, with the heel of your hand on one side and your fingertips on the other side of the ropy muscles. Gradually squeeze until the pressure is comfortable, making contact with the B 10 points. Gently place the fingertips and thumb of your left hand on GB 14 (on your forehead, one finger-width above the eyebrows, in line with the pupils). Hold this point combination for two minutes while breathing deeply.

Step 2

Hold B 10 with St 3: Move your left hand to St 3 (below your cheekbone) and gently angle your pressure upward. Breathe deeply for two minutes. Continue to hold your neck with your right hand.

Step 3

Hold B 10 with CV 17: Place your left hand on CV 17 (at the center of the breastbone, at heart level). Feel for the indentations in the bone, using all of your fingertips to hold the hollow spaces. Your right hand continues to squeeze your neck muscles firmly. As you hold this position, close your eyes, and take long, slow, deep breaths into your heart for two minutes.

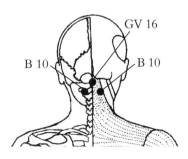

GV 16

B 10   B 10

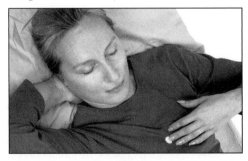

Step 4

Hold GV 16 with Three Points: Reposition your right middle finger on GV 16 (in the center hollow at the base of your skull). Tilt your head back slowly and comfortably. Apply firm pressure into GV 16, angling into the center of your head. Keep your right hand at the base of the skull as you place your left hand in the following positions:

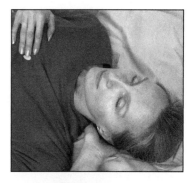

- **Center of the Breastbone (CV 17):** As you continue to hold CV 17 at the center of the breastbone, take several deep breaths into your belly for two minutes. As you inhale, visualize breathing into what you are worrying about. Then exhale your worries away.

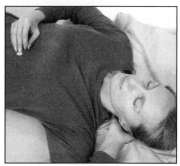

- **Base of Ribcage (Sp 16):** Apply gentle pressure on Sp 16 (at the base of your ribcage); use your fingertips on the right side and the heel of your hand on the left side. This balances the energy flows for a person who worries excessively. Breathe deeply into your stomach for two minutes. Visualize your worry being released.

- **Center of Belly (CV 12):** Move your left hand an inch down, placing the palm of your hand firmly over your stomach. Concentrate on breathing deeply into your stomach for two minutes. Tell yourself to just relax. Affirm in your mind there is nothing worth losing your balance over.

Step 5

Deeply Relax, Palming CV 6: Place your hands two finger-widths below the navel to palm CV 6. Close your eyes, and continue to breathe deeply. Remind yourself that there is nothing worth worrying about. Let yourself completely relax for the next ten minutes.

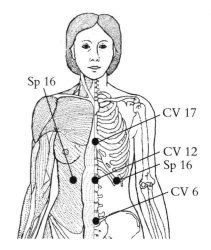

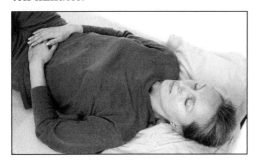

PART III:

PHYSICAL
IMBALANCES

Ninety percent of all physical problems have psychological roots.... A growing body of evidence indicates that virtually every ill that can befall the body—from acne to arthritis, headaches to heart disease, cold sores to cancer—is influenced, for better or worse, by our emotions.

— Emrika Padus, Editor
The Complete Guide to Your Emotions & Your Health

22
CHRONIC FATIGUE & FIBROMYALGIA

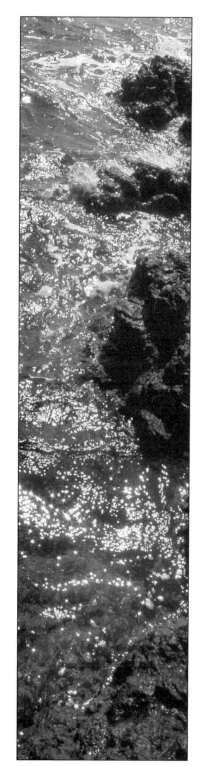

Chronic fatigue syndrome and fibromyalgia are rooted in similar immune system abnormalities. Both conditions have the following overlapping symptoms: headache, aching muscles, soreness, sleep disturbances, joint swelling, irritable bowel syndrome, food allergies, hypersensitivity to weather conditions, environmental stress, confusion, and emotional imbalances. Muscle pain is the primary complaint of fibromyalgia, whereas chronic fatigue sufferers complain predominantly about feeling exhausted. Both chronic fatigue and fibromyalgia can cause the onset of viral infections, retroviruses, and excess yeast in the system. Antibiotics, chemical toxins, thyroid and steroid medications, oral contraceptives, and hereditary disorders can exacerbate the symptoms of these conditions.

By working with chronic fatigue and fibromyalgia, we have discovered a connection between immune system functions, emotional stress, and trauma. We have applied this insight to many other emotional problems. People with either chronic fatigue or fibromyalgia have often suffered from traumatic experiences that virtually shut down the immune system. Not everyone who has experienced trauma is struck with chronic fatigue or fibromyalgia—many people are resistant to illnesses due to their inherited constitution, while others are fortunate enough to receive the attention necessary to heal after a traumatic event. But millions who are jolted inside continue to suffer from chronic fatigue or fibromyalgia. We have discovered ways to use acupressure that have enabled many people with these conditions to release their trauma, heal significantly, and even reduce their drug therapy.

The immune system is designed to fight off anything it perceives as a threat. Under normal conditions, it fights off an attack

Affirmations to Counteract Chronic Fatigue & Fibromyalgia

• *Each deep breath I take decreases my pain.*

• *Healing energy is flowing through my body.*

• *I am letting go of my past traumas.*

• *I am strengthening my body by breathing deeply.*

• *I listen to the messages of my body for healing myself.*

and then relaxes. But in both chronic fatigue and fibromyalgia, the immune system continues to act as though it is under attack long after the disturbance has passed. This can trigger multiple emotional reactions, such as excessive worry, fear, or overwhelming emotion that can further deplete the body's energy reserves and weaken the immune system. Since most traumatic experiences are unresolved, the immune system continues to be taxed.

The link we discovered was enlightening; although the stories our clients and students told us were different, the common thread was the same for those with chronic fatigue and fibromyalgia. Anyone with a history involving trauma, whether from an accident or a severe emotional upset, became more susceptible to chronic fatigue and fibromyalgia due to a weakened immune system.

Kathleen was an active middle-aged wife and mother. She worked part time, loved to travel, enjoyed her children, and generally had a zest for life. All of this changed after a routine breast exam turned into a nightmare.

During the exam Kathleen told the nurse the pressure was too much, the pain to her breast was excruciating. After having had an exam routinely every year, she knew something wasn't right. The nurse told Kathleen, "Stop being such a baby. You are old enough to tolerate a little discomfort." Kathleen recalled her anger and devastation. When she left the hospital, she was unable to lift her right arm. The next day her breast tissue had swollen to twice its normal size and was completely black and blue. She went from doctor to doctor for a year trying to get relief from the pain. No one in the medical community helped her sort out this traumatic experience. They offered medication, physical therapy, and biofeedback, all of which were of only temporary help.

A year after the exam Kathleen was diagnosed with chronic fatigue syndrome. The debilitating fatigue forced her to quit her job and end all social activities with her family and friends. When she met Beth Henning, all she could do was lie on the couch and pray that her pain would disappear.

Kathleen often cried during her acupressure sessions, saying she felt she had been deeply violated and abused by her health care providers. She had trusted her routine exams to prevent major medical problems. Her experience with the mammogram technician completely changed that trust.

Beth taught the following self-help routines to Kathleen's husband, who faithfully applied them every day. Within four weeks Kathleen was able to do the point sequences on her own. By listening to her body's emotional cues, Kathleen was able to achieve balance again.

After five months of daily self-help, she began teaching the points she had learned to her local chronic fatigue group. She continues to share her excitement about using self-acupressure and is extremely grateful for regaining her vitality.

DIETARY CONSIDERATIONS

Chronic fatigue and fibromyalgia often tax the body's ability to digest food; many people suddenly find their body reacting negatively to many foods that were never a problem before. Dietary changes can therefore be an important part of recovery. Experiment with the following suggestions and apply whatever you find useful.

- **Decrease or Eliminate Dairy Products:** Dairy products are mucus forming and can cause congestion. Bacteria within your body can fester and is more prevalent when the body is congested. So minimize your consumption of dairy products.

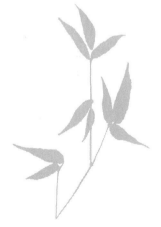

- **Decrease Cold & Raw Foods:** If you suffer from chronic fatigue or fibromyalgia these foods will strain your system. Eat lightly steamed or sautéed vegetables rather than raw foods.

- **Increase Greens:** Leafy greens such as collards, kale, Swiss chard, spinach (but eat spinach sparingly if osteoporosis is present), Chinese cabbage, and mustard greens will increase your vitality and boost your immune system.

- **Eat Sea Vegetables:** Adding seaweed to soups, vegetables, and grains is an excellent way to obtain valuable trace minerals and vitamins naturally.

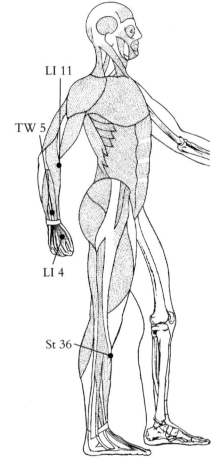

LI 11

TW 5

LI 4

St 36

- **Reduce Wheat & Yeast Products:** Pay attention to how your body feels after eating these foods—they often cause allergic reactions. Toasting bread helps your body digest and break down the yeast-wheat-sugar combination. You can find gluten-free or yeast-free cookbooks and yeast-free breads at your local health food store. Try making gluten-free bread at home.

- **Eliminate Sugar:** Eliminate white sugar products completely from your diet. Replace them with more wholesome sweet foods such as yams, squash, apples, and carrots. When baking, try replacing white sugar and honey with 100 percent pure apple juice.

- **Eat Fruit Moderately:** Since fruit contains a lot of sugar, moderation is necessary. Citrus and tropical fruits are especially high in sugar and are acidic. Combining fruits and vegetables during a meal can cause digestive imbalances. Eat fruit by itself as a healthy snack.

- **Eliminate Caffeine, Sodas & Alcohol:** Consuming alcohol and caffeine can suppress the immune system. Drinking a lot of coffee daily can be a factor in sluggishness and depression. The oils and residue of the coffee bean, found even in decaffeinated coffee, can tax the immune system. Try replacing coffee with green teas, which contain smaller amounts of caffeine, herbal teas, or grain-based drinks such as roasted barley.

- **Get Enough Protein:** Make sure you get adequate protein on a daily basis. Two to four ounces of good-quality protein foods can rebuild your body's vital energy. Use organic foods when possible, to obtain more nutrients and to avoid the intake of poisonous pesticides and harmful hormones.

- **Take Baths:** Ginger baths are revitalizing to the digestive system and relieve achy, stiff muscles. Place a quarter-cup fresh-grated ginger root in cheesecloth, nylon, or other porous material and set it directly in the bathtub. Soak your body for fifteen minutes in the hot bath. Take a brief nap afterward.

QUICK TIPS FOR
CHRONIC FATIGUE & FIBROMYALGIA

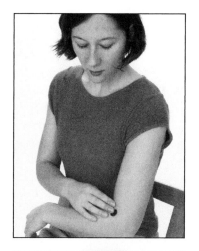

For optimum relief from chronic fatigue and fibromyalgia symptoms, practice self-acupressure daily. The following bilateral points benefit the immune system. You do not have to use all of them; one or two alone can be effective.

Be sure to apply and release your finger pressure slowly when working to heal sore muscles and tissues. Gradually increase the pressure and amount of time you spend on a point. Go slowly and use less pressure to avoid aggravating your body's tenderness; the effects of acupressure can be strong.

LI 11 (on the outside of the arm, at the end of the elbow crease): Bend your arm to feel where the bones meet in a V shape. Apply firm pressure into the joint. Hold for two minutes, to fortify the immune system.

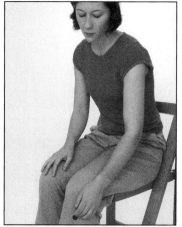

St 36 (one palm-width below the kneecap, between the tendons of the outer legs): This point is useful for fatigue, endurance, and improving digestion. Use steady, firm pressure to hold this point for two minutes. Whenever your energy is low, try briskly rubbing St 36. This is excellent to do at work, while riding the bus, or sitting anywhere for a long period of time.

Index Finger: Grasp each index finger firmly (one at a time) for two minutes, until you feel a smooth, steady pulse. Breathe deeply into your abdomen and tell yourself to simply relax.

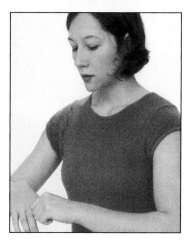

LI 4 (in the webbing between the thumb and index finger): Apply firm pressure into the angle of the bones. Holding this point is particularly beneficial for pain relief, inflammation, sluggish elimination, moodiness, headaches, flu-like symptoms, and food sensitivities.

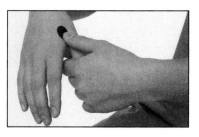

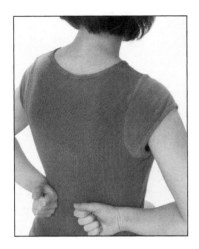

MINIROUTINES FOR
CHRONIC FATIGUE & FIBROMYALGIA

Rub Lower Back gently but briskly with the palms of both hands at waist level: If you are extremely sore, simply hold your lower back instead of rubbing. This stimulates the Sea of Vitality points (B 23, B 47), revitalizing the entire body.

Hold Third Eye with Sea of Tranquility: Place the right hand on the center of the breastbone (CV 17) and the left hand on the Third Eye point (GV 24.5) between the brows. Breathe deeply into your abdomen for one to three minutes, to release stress and tension.

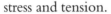

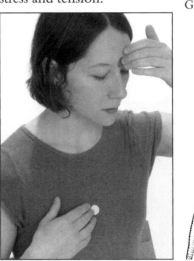

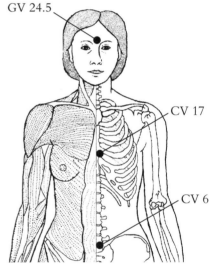

GV 24.5

CV 17

CV 6

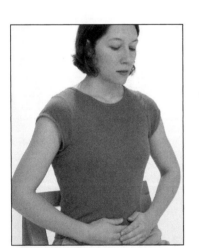

Palm Lower Abdomen: Place the palms of both hands three finger-widths below your navel. Pressing this powerful tonic point (CV 6) strengthens the entire body. For best results, use deep abdominal breathing and healing affirmations as you hold this point for one to three minutes.

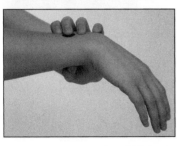

Hold Inner & Outer Wrist: Place your middle finger on the outside and your thumb on the inside of your wrist, two to three finger-widths from the wrist crease, to hold P 6 with TW 5. Allow your hand to rest comfortably on your lap with your eyes closed as you continue to hold these balancing points in a relaxed position for two minutes. Then switch to work on the other side for two more minutes.

SELF-CARE ROUTINE FOR
CHRONIC FATIGUE & FIBROMYALGIA

This routine helps to alleviate the worry, fear, and back pain associated with chronic fatigue and fibromyalgia. Use deep abdominal breathing to increase circulation to every part of your body. Sit up in a comfortable position; have a blanket nearby for the deep relaxation afterward. If your time is limited, you do not have to use all of these points to be effective—using just one or two while breathing deeply can be beneficial to relieving stress.

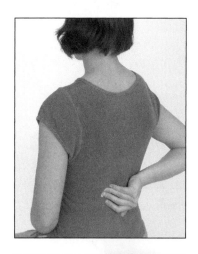

Step 1

Hold Lower Back (B 47): Notice which side of your body feels tighter, and work on that side. If your right side feels tighter, use your right hand to hold the right B 47. If your left side feels tighter, use your left hand to hold the left B 47. This point, on the lower back, is at waist level on the thick ropy muscles, two to four finger-widths away from the spine. Your hand will stay in this position as you go on to the next steps.

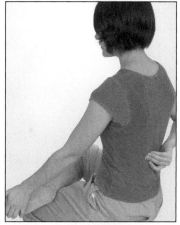

Step 2

Hold Lower Back and the Big Toe: Continue to hold the tighter side of your lower back. Cross your leg, bringing your foot onto your thigh, and grasp the big toe to stimulate the points at the base of the nail. As you hold these points, focus on your breath for one minute. If your thoughts start to wander, bring your awareness back into your fingertips, to heighten the flow of healing energy.

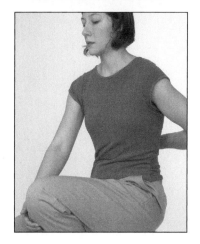

Step 3

Hold Lower Back and St 36: Move the hand holding your big toe up your leg to St 36 (located on the outside of the leg, one palm-width below the knee). Breathe deeply for two minutes as you hold these points to increase healing energy for the immune system.

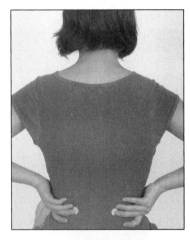

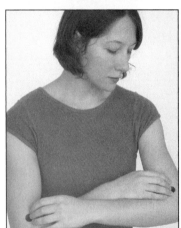

Step 4

Hold the Lower Back (B 47): Using both hands, place your fingertips on the ropy muscles in your lower back at waist level, four finger-widths out from the spine. Focus on your breath for two minutes, to deepen your body awareness and imagine increased healing energy circulating to each cell as your hands radiate heat into your lower back.

Step 5

Hold Opposite LI 11s: Cross your forearms to reach the opposite elbow crease on the outside of each arm. Using your fingertips, apply moderate to firm pressure on LI 11. Affirm your body's ability to heal as you breathe into your abdomen for one minute.

Step 6

Deep Relaxation: Completely relax for five to fifteen minutes in a comfortable position, to reap all the benefits.

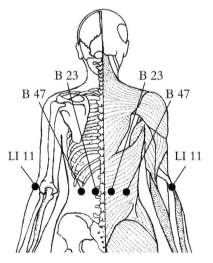

23

INSOMNIA

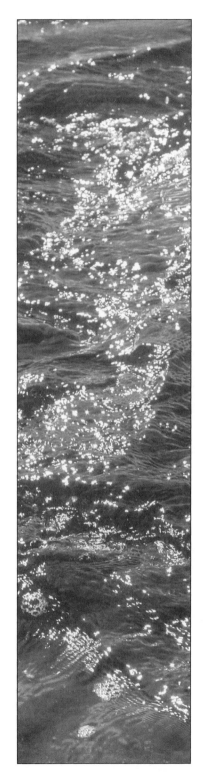

Many people find it hard to fall asleep when they have something troubling on their minds. Getting a good night's rest can seem impossible when you are experiencing run-of-the-mill frustrations or anxieties or are just plain stressed out. Obsessive thoughts and images of unresolved trauma can fill your mind with memories that simply won't quiet down. The shock from an accident or violent episode can cause the body's muscles to contract and remain tense long after the event. Chronic tension and physical pain cause insomnia, as can a host of medical problems like arthritis and heart disease. Emotional and behavioral problems such as repressed or blocked motivation, frustration, apathy, depression, worry, or anxiety further exacerbate sleeping disorders.

The inability to get to sleep, or stay asleep, can be caused also by noise, sexual frustration, medication side effects, changes in schedule, or a nighttime work schedule. Smoking, eating, drinking alcohol, and especially drinking caffeine before bedtime can also cause insomnia.

Throughout this book we've looked at how emotions become rooted in the body. Anxiety is often rooted in the upper back and chest muscles. Hurt from divorce or betrayal causes knots of tension between the shoulder blades. Holding acupressure points can release upper body tension and relieve insomnia at the same time.

There are many types of insomnia. In addition to trouble getting to sleep, it can also mean problems such as waking up frequently during the night with trouble returning to sleep, awakening too early in the morning, and sleep that is not refreshing, that is, feeling like you didn't get enough sleep.

Some sleep problem patterns may be caused by a blockage in the meridian that flows through predominantly at the time when a person either can't get to sleep or awakens too soon. For instance, if a person feels energetic, inspired, or hyped-up and cannot get to sleep between eleven P.M. and one A.M., it may indicate that frustration is jamming the Gall Bladder meridian.

But if a person has repressed anger, or has a tendency to eat a lot of rich, oily, high-cholesterol foods such as butter and French fries, his or her Liver meridian may be congested, which will cause sleep disturbances between one and three in the morning.

People with grief issues and difficulty letting go may have blockages in their Lung meridian and thus may wake up between three and five in the morning.

Dealing with the emotion associated with the meridian that is imbalanced, and getting enough exercise—particularly stretching and aerobic exercise—will not only open the meridian but also work out the tension that can contribute to insomnia.

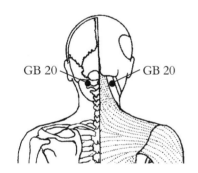

GB 20   GB 20

Jody, a recent divorcée, suffered from insomnia for several months. She had not slept well since her husband verbally abused her in the last days of their marriage. She was going through the divorce and caring for her three children on her own. Behind her polite smile she looked exhausted.

Michael Gach showed Jody how to work on acupressure points under the base of the skull (GB 20) and on both sides of each ankle (K 6, B 62) to relieve her sleep disorders. Spirit Gate (H 7, located on the inside of the wrist below the little finger) and Inner Gate (P 6, located on the center of the inner wrist, three finger-widths above the wrist crease) balanced and calmed her heart. Jody used these points on a regular daily basis and reported deeper, undisturbed sleep and more alertness. In addition, holding these points alleviated her anxiety, harmonized her emotional stress, and nurtured her spiritual awareness.

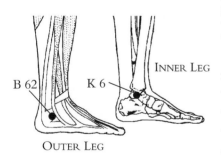

INNER LEG

B 62   K 6

OUTER LEG

Michael also gave Jody a gentle relaxation program to do before going to bed. He recommended that she give up coffee and try hot water with lemon, Roast Aroma, or ginger tea. Within three weeks Jody called to say she hadn't slept so soundly in years. She continued her daily practice and hasn't touched a drop of caffeine since.

Dietary Considerations

Caffeine is a well-known stimulant and a major culprit in sleeping disorders. Coffee, soft drinks, and black teas contain caffeine, which can keep you up at night. If you have any complaints about sleeping, cut out caffeine permanently, or at least several hours before bedtime.

Foods high in saturated fat and cholesterol can also cause insomnia. As the blood carries these fatty deposits, they attach to the walls of the blood vessels. This narrows the passageways and makes the heart work harder to pump the blood. In traditional Chinese medicine, stress on the heart is known to affect a person's emotional well-being and ability to sleep.

Eating before going to bed can also create insomnia. The food speeds up your metabolism; sleep slows it down. Your metabolism is getting two opposite, conflicting messages. This conflict creates wear and tear on the body and commonly causes horrible nightmares.

QUICK TIPS FOR INSOMNIA

The following suggestions can help you relax and get to sleep.

Yawning & Stretching: Exaggerate several yawns as you stretch out your arms, back, and legs. This relaxes your body and increases the circulation in preparation for getting to sleep.

Slow, Deep Breathing: Concentrate on breathing deeply into your belly. Slow, deep breathing calms your emotions and instantly relaxes your body.

Eye-Stretching Exercises: With your eyes open, move your eyes in a large circle around the periphery of your vision three times in each direction. Repeat this eye rotation with your eyes closed as you focus on your breath. End by inducing a few yawns as you stretch your arms up and out.

Affirmations to Counteract Insomnia

- *I love to go to sleep.*

- *I release and let go.*

- *I am at peace with myself.*

- *I feel safe, comfortable, and cozy.*

- *I enjoy feeling how my whole body relaxes when I get into bed.*

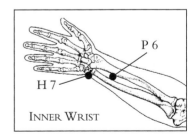

P 6

H 7

INNER WRIST

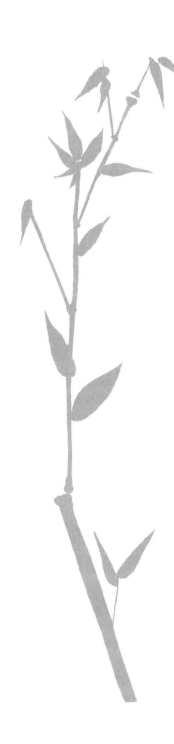

Deep Relaxation: Lie down comfortably on your back or side, and gently close your eyes. Take long, slow, deep breaths as you tell each part of your body to completely relax. Begin with your feet and legs, slowly moving up toward your head. With each exhalation, completely relax whatever part of the body you are focusing on. Let your mind be clear of any extraneous thoughts, and meditate on breathing deeply and relaxing every cell of your body.

Hot Baths: Use candles, essential oils, and soft music to set the stage for your healing. Placing a half-cup of sea salt, a half-cup of baking soda, and a few drops of essential oil (lavender is very soothing) in your bathwater is an effective replacement for expensive mineral salts and fragrance combinations. Deep breathing, stretching, and a hot bath are healing and deeply relaxing after an emotional trauma.

Herbal Teas: Taking chamomile tea before bedtime can encourage deep sleep. Chamomile is gentle and very safe for adults as well as children. To make the tea, boil two cups of water and remove from heat. Add a quarter-cup of the dried herb, and let the mixture steep for fifteen minutes, producing a warm yellow tea. Strain the mixture and serve. Chamomile added into children's fruit juice or a warmed beverage encourages deep, relaxing sleep.

Yoga: Refer to Part III under Insomnia in the book *Acu-Yoga,* by Michael Reed Gach, Japan Publications, for yogic practices, breathing meditations, and stretching to promote sound sleep.

ACUPRESSURE POINTS
FOR RELIEVING INSOMNIA

H 7 (Spirit Gate, located on the inside of the wrist crease, in line with the little finger): Holding H 7 relieves anxiety and insomnia due to overexcitement.

B 10 (Heavenly Pillar, located a half-inch below the base of the skull, on the ropy muscles, and a half-inch outward from the spine): Holding B 10 relieves stress, burnout, insomnia, irritability, exhaustion, stiff neck, repressed anger, resentment, and sore throat.

GB 20 (Gates of Consciousness, located below the base of the skull, in the hollows between the two large vertical neck muscles, two or three inches apart depending on the size of the head): Holding GB 20 relieves arthritis in the shoulders and neck, headaches, mental stress, frustration, anger, and other aches and pains that contribute to insomnia.

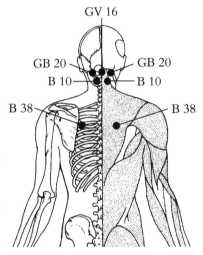

B 38 (Vital Diaphragm, located between the shoulder blades and the spine, at the level of the heart): Holding B 38 relieves insomnia, enhances breathing, calms anxiety, and is a good emotional balancing point.

GV 16 (Wind Mansion, located in the center of the back of the head, in a large hollow under the base of the skull): Holding GV 16 relieves insomnia, headaches, general overall body pain, and mental stress.

P 6 (Inner Gate, located in the middle of the inside of the forearm, two and a half finger-widths from the wrist crease): Holding P 6 relieves insomnia, anxiety, anger, agitation, nausea, hiccups, chest pain, palpitations, other emotional imbalances, shock, dizziness, and trauma.

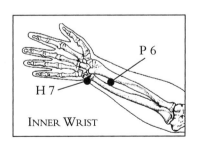

INNER WRIST

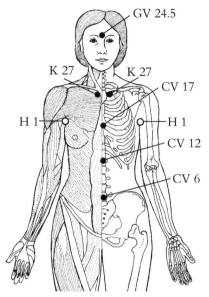

GV 24.5

K 27   K 27

H 1   CV 17   H 1

CV 12

CV 6

○ – H 1 is in the center
of the armpit.

GV 24.5 (Third Eye, located between the eyebrows, in the indentation where the bridge of the nose meets the forehead): Holding GV 24.5 balances the pituitary gland and relaxes the central nervous system for relieving anxiety and insomnia.

CV 17 (Sea of Tranquility, located on the center of the breastbone, four finger-widths up from the base of the bone): Holding CV 17 relieves nervousness, emotional uptightness, and anxiety that can cause insomnia.

K 6 (Joyful Sleep, located directly below the inside of the anklebone, in a slight indentation): Holding K 6 relieves insomnia, heel and ankle pain, hypertension, and anxiety.

B 62 (Calm Sleep, located in the first indentation directly below the outer anklebone): Holding B 62 relieves insomnia and the back pain that makes it difficult to sleep.

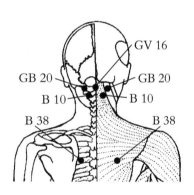

GV 16

GB 20   GB 20

B 10   B 10

B 38   B 38

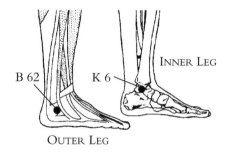

INNER LEG

B 62   K 6

OUTER LEG

QUICK TIPS FOR
INSOMNIA

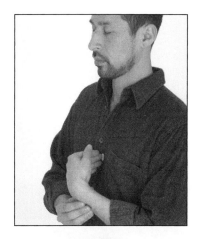

Hold P 6 & TW 5 with CV 17: Grasp these wrist points (located three finger-widths from the wrist crease, on the inner and outer arm) with your thumb and fingertip. Use the outside knuckle of your thumb to press CV 17 (at the center of the chest). Holding these points while breathing deeply for two or three minutes can soothe an emotional upset.

Touch CV 6 with CV 12: Press CV 6 (in the lower belly) with your right hand and CV 12 (in the center of the abdomen) with your left hand. Inhale deeply as you visualize healing energy coming up the back of your legs through your spine, up to the top of your head. Hold your breath for a second or two. Exhale, and imagine the energy flowing down your face through your body, ending at the tips of your toes. Practice this breathing meditation while sitting, standing, or lying down comfortably on your back for three minutes, to relieve abdominal pain, poor eating habits, insomnia, and emotional stress.

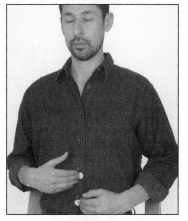

Hold K 27 with GV 16: Place your right fingertips into GV 16 (at the base of the skull). Use your left thumb and fingers to hold K 27 (on both sides, below the head of the collarbones, in the hollow spaces), and breathe deeply for two minutes. Holding these points together harmonizes thoughts as well as the energy flow through the upper back, shoulders, and neck.

Hold H 1 with Opposite Hands: Cross your hands over your chest to reach the H 1 points (in the middle of your armpits). Holding these emotional balancing points harmonizes spiritual unrest. Breathe deeply, and tell yourself to relax as you hold these points for one minute.

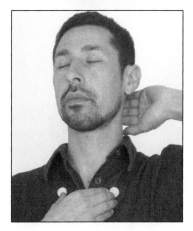

SELF-CARE FOR
INSOMNIA*

The following self-care routine is most effective when done lying down, but (except for step 1) you can also practice it sitting comfortably. Help prevent and relieve insomnia by following these instructions:

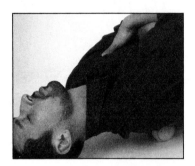

Step 1

Use Tennis Balls to Press B 38: Lie down on two tennis balls, placing them in between your shoulder blades. Close your eyes, and breathe deeply for one minute.

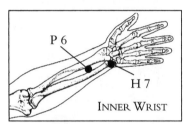

Step 2

Press P 6: Place your right thumb on the inside of your left wrist with your fingers directly behind, three finger-widths from the wrist crease. Press firmly for one minute. Then switch sides to press the point on your other wrist.

P 6

H 7

INNER WRIST

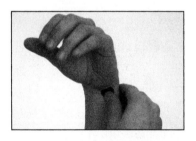

Step 3

Hold H 7: Place your right thumb or fingers on the inside wrist crease of your left hand, directly below your little finger. Feel for a hollow to press Spirit Gate (H 7). After holding for one minute, switch sides to hold the point on your right wrist for one minute as you breathe deeply.

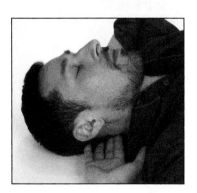

Step 4

Firmly Press B 10: Curve your fingers, placing your fingertips on the thick, ropy muscles on the back of your neck. Apply firm pressure as you breathe deeply for two minutes.

---

*For insomnia relief we suggest the following guided self-healing audio CD: Michael Reed Gach, *Sleep Better* (Sounds True, 2003).

Step 5

Press GV 16: Place your middle fingers in the large hollow at the center of the base of your skull. Close your eyes, slowly tilt your head back, and breathe deeply as you press firmly into this hollow area for one minute. Induce yawning while breathing into this point to help you get to sleep.

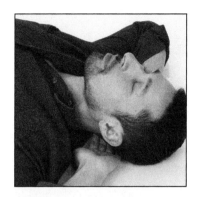

Step 6

Press up into GB 20: Use your thumbs to gradually press underneath the base of your skull, about three inches apart. Keeping your eyes closed, slowly tilt your head back as you use your thumbs to firmly press up and underneath your skull for one minute or until you feel a regular, even pulse on both sides.

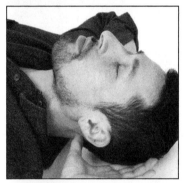

Step 7

Hold GV 24.5 along with CV 17: Place your right middle fingertip in between your eyebrows in the indentation between the bridge of your nose and your forehead. Position the fingertips of your left hand on CV 17 (in the indentations of your breastbone, at the level of your heart). With your eyes closed, apply steady, firm pressure, and breathe deeply for one minute.

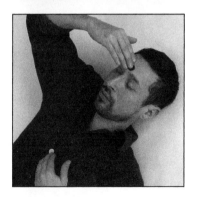

Step 8

Hold K 6 with B 62: Use your thumbs to hold the K 6 points (on the inside of each ankle in the indentations below the inner anklebone). Position your fingertips directly across from your thumb, on the other side of your anklebone, to press B 62, (directly below the outer anklebone). Hold these points for one minute as you breathe deeply to relieve insomnia.

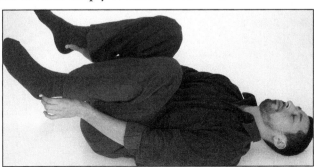

24

MENSTRUATION & MENOPAUSE

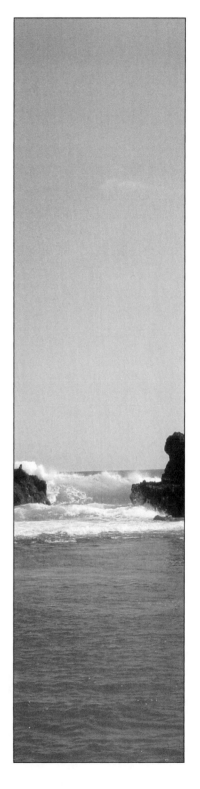

A cupressure balances the hormonal system and empowers women to reclaim the natural rhythm of their cycles. When a woman's hormones change, tremendous emotional upheavals often occur. Acupressure can be useful for reducing the stress and balancing the emotions during puberty, menstruation, perimenopause, and menopause. Customized self-acupressure can harmonize a woman's unique body chemistry, relieve symptoms, and support a balanced diet and lifestyle. Acupressure has no harmful side effects and can be self-administered without expensive equipment.

Self-acupressure increases women's ability to manage stress; daily practice can keep the body in balance. Emotional stress, coupled with painful symptoms, distract women from appreciating their internal rhythms and their bond with creation. The nurturing touch of acupressure can also strengthen a woman's awareness of her cycles and harmonize the endocrine system.

Premenstrual Syndrome (PMS)

PMS symptoms, which occur one to two weeks prior to the onset of menstruation, include irritability, anger, hypersensitivity, mood swings, withdrawal, headaches, food cravings, and bloating. Emotional upset often lengthens the duration of PMS. Women with a history of trauma and abuse can suffer from PMS all month long. Women are more vulnerable to PMS symptoms if their tensions and painful memories are not processed and released.

For instance, the issues and feelings involved in the sudden ending of an intimate relationship can often interrupt a woman's cycle. The grief of letting go and fear of the unknown can create hormonal imbalances and tremendous stress. Women need time to explore their unresolved issues, to transform old patterns, and to heal emotional wounds. Cycle irregularities and increased symptoms can be an intuitive signal from a woman's body to slow down, breathe deeply, and obtain healing support.

After learning of her husband's infidelity, Cindy suffered with PMS symptoms for three out of four weeks of the month. The stress, anger, and worry of this betrayal resulted in physical ailments such as lower back pain and headaches. Just before her menstruation, she was extremely depressed and agitated. At the onset of menstruation, pain would shoot through her legs and pelvis, making her work unbearable. Medications did not change her PMS symptoms. A regimen combining acupressure, exercise, deep relaxation, stretching, and conscious dietary change was essential to Cindy's emotional stability.

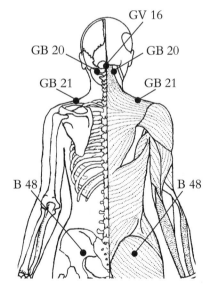

Stacy, at twenty-two, was suffering from severe PMS. Her migraine headaches and deep mood swings occurred during ovulation. Sugar and salt cravings caused body soreness and swelling. Neck pain kept her home from work one day per month. Cramping and heavy bleeding would not diminish, despite the birth control pills and antidepressants her doctors prescribed.

Stacy's symptoms increased after she broke up with her boyfriend. She moved across the country to be with him, only to find he really didn't love her. She was devastated and shocked. The emotional stress magnified her PMS symptoms.

Several points helped Stacy gently let go of the man she loved. Holding the shoulder and neck points GB 21, GB 20, and GV 16 relieved her muscle tension, worry, infatuation, and mental stress. Holding the groin and leg points CV 6, Sp 12, Sp 13, and Sp 10 relieved the anger, frustration, and tension in her pelvic area. Holding the heart and chest points CV 17, Lu 1, and K 27 released tears and deep feelings of abandonment and resentment. Reliving rather then avoiding her emotions became a milestone for resolving Stacy's PMS symptoms.

Stacy's self-care included stretching, acupressure, and deep relaxation. She also learned to manage her food cravings. After six months of consciously working with her cycle, she was pain free. Her symptoms have not returned, and she continues to practice self-acupressure on a regular basis.

DIETARY & LIFESTYLE CONSIDERATIONS

Reduce the following:

- dairy consumption
- caffeine, white sugar, soft drinks, and chocolate
- butter and animal fat (good alternatives are sesame, olive, and safflower oils)

Increase the following:

- whole grains and fresh vegetables
- exercise, stretching, and deep relaxation

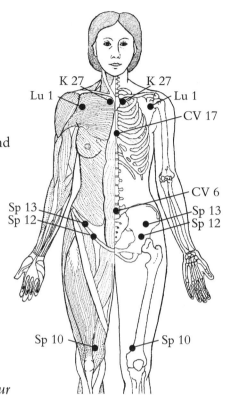

SELF-CARE ROUTINE FOR PMS

Create a safe, healing environment. Wear loose clothing so your body can move freely. Begin this acupressure routine by lying comfortably on your back.

Step 1

Roll on B 48: Stimulate the sacral points by lying on your back and placing your fists on B 48 (beside the base of the spine). Gently roll from side to side for one minute. Move your fists two inches outward and down slightly. Roll from side to side for another minute. This exercise releases emotional stress and tension in the pelvis and buttocks associated with menstrual cramps and PMS symptoms.

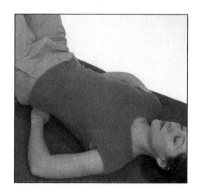

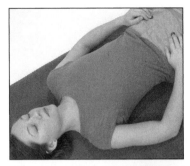

Step 2

Hold Sp 12 & Sp 13: Hold these points with your fingertips (in the middle of the crease where the leg joins the trunk of the body). This reduces frustration, bloating, and cramping. Breathe deeply into your belly for two minutes. Image a golden cord of healing energy moving through your pelvis and legs, linking you to the earth.

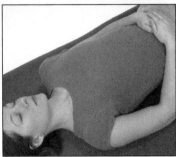

Step 3

Hold CV 6 (three finger-widths below your navel): Slowly apply firm palm pressure as you breathe deeply into your belly for two minutes. Continue to imagine a warm, golden cord originating from this point through your legs and going into the soles of your feet. Feel the warmth of this energy nourishing you.

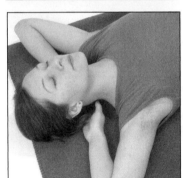

Step 4

Hold GB 20: Place your fingertips into the hollow spaces below the skull. Apply gentle traction as you tilt your head back. Relax your shoulders and breathe deeply for one minute.

Step 5

Hold GV 20 with GV 24.5: Place one hand on GV 20 (at the crown of your head) and the other on GV 24.5 (at the center brow point). Inhale deeply, taking in healing energy. As you exhale, breathe out any mental stress or tension for two minutes.

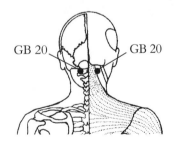

GB 20   GB 20

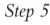

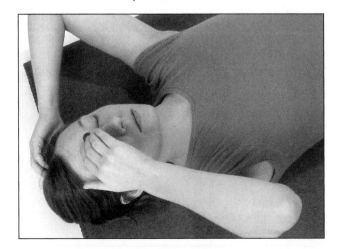

Step 6

Hold CV 17: Palm the center of the breastbone by placing one hand over the other for two minutes. Breathe deeply as you pay attention to the circulation of healing energy flowing through your body. Tell yourself to completely relax as you explore any body sensations or feelings.

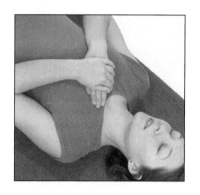

Step 7

Deep Relaxation: Place your hands at your sides, and relax deeply for five minutes. An herbal bath can be a wonderful way to rest after your self-care session.

Menstruation

Most young women begin menstruation in their early teens. Exercise, diet, stress, and genetics play a major role in menstrual onset and regularity. The number of eggs a woman is born with can determine how long she is fertile.

Ovulation occurs in midcycle, when a woman's egg can become fertilized. If the egg is not fertilized, menstruation will begin approximately fourteen days later. Hormones govern the interaction between the hypothalamus, the ovaries, and the pituitary gland, significantly influencing the quality of a woman's emotional life.

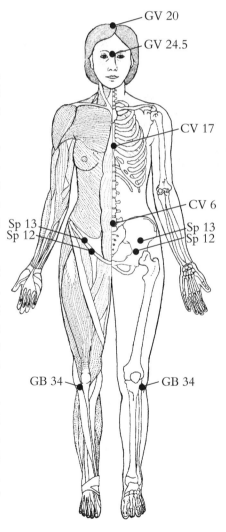

Sara was twelve and had just begun her period. Her mother wanted her to celebrate this event rather than view it as a burden. Sara felt a little embarrassed by her enthusiasm and did not want to invite any of her friends. Instead, she invited eight women friends of Sara's and her family to the celebration. Everyone was asked to share a story and bring a gift to signify Sara's transition to womanhood.

Beth's gift was to teach Sara herbs and self-acupressure for relaxing and balancing her body during menstruation. She learned Sp 12, Sp 13, Sp 6, Sp 10, CV 6, GB 34, and an acupressure self-hug. In addition, the women went to Beth's garden and gathered chamomile for relaxation, raspberry leaf to tone and strengthen her uterus, and lavender and mint for a hot herbal bath. Other women shared songs, birthing tales, and first sexual experiences. They laughed, cried, and played together for hours.

Affirmations for Menstruation

• *I am open to the wide range of feelings I go through each month.*

• *My body's cycles are sacred.*

• *I am breathing deeply, appreciating my body's wisdom.*

• *I am in touch with the healing energy of my body.*

• *My menstrual cycle heightens my awareness.*

In the afternoon, the group of women took Sara to the mall to buy nail polish, soap, natural scents and oils, candles and a bouquet of flowers. She picked her favorite place for the group to have lunch together. The celebration ended by swimming at the beach and standing in a circle holding hands around a fire. Each woman prayed and affirmed a special blessing for Sara. Collectively the women promised to offer ongoing guidance and support in answering any questions she would have about womanhood.

Now seventeen, Sara has no negative PMS symptoms. She exercises, uses self-acupressure and herbs as prevention, and rests when she feels stressed or tired. She embraces her cycle by listening to her body and the natural rhythm of her emotions. Although she was a little embarrassed about her party at the time, she looks back on that day as a beautiful expression of her mother's love. She has already thought of ways to create a similar celebration for her young nieces.

Menstruation is a time for silence, reflection, and prayer. The desire to go inward, withdrawing from social activities and personal relationships, is part of the natural rhythm. Most women need more time for rest and solitude during menstruation. Take this time to nourish yourself and listen to your inner needs.

Journaling

Journaling has helped many women track the beauty and wonder of their cycle. Writing down feelings and cravings in relationship to menstruation helps women be more conscious. When they record what part of their moon cycle generates breast tenderness, cramping, libido levels, and irritability, they often begin to have empowering insights. Women can regulate their symptoms by creatively designing a home acupressure program.

Charting your menstrual cycle can be a worthwhile practice. Start by creating a calendar that lists thirty days across the top. If your cycle is longer than thirty days, add as many more as you need. Make a list of your menstrual symptoms on the left-hand side, to create a graph. Put a check under the day of the month when the symptom occurred. For example, you might list food cravings, mood swings, anxiety, and menstrual cramps, just to name a few. Add the moon phases if your symptoms seem sporadic and unidentifiable. Often mood swings, food cravings, and body pain occur at a particular moon phase in relation to a woman's cycle. Knowing this helps women plan their monthly activities.

Mark an M in the box for the first day of menstruation. Continue filling in your chart daily and marking the level of severity of your symptoms. Use a rating ratio of one to five, five being the most severe. If you are feeling in balance, leave the box empty. In addition, leave additional lines somewhere on the calendar to jot down emotional triggers and your daily reactions.

You can also develop a more complicated charting system to record the consistency of your vaginal discharge over each month. Different stages of mucus are produced during each part of a woman's cycle. This discharge peaks at ovulation and minimizes after a woman's period. Many traditions use this mucus identification as a "rhythm method," effective for natural birth control and fertility awareness. Check your local women's center or public library for more information on natural birth control and charting.

After a couple of months of charting their cycle and journaling, many women have discovered the relationship between their hormones, feelings, and actions. We encourage you to explore this beneficial practice to increase your awareness and emotional balance.

SELF-CARE ROUTINE FOR MENSTRUATION

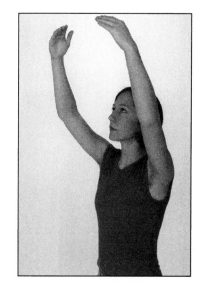

For this self-care routine, wear comfortable, loose clothing. Be sure to have pillows and a blanket available during the mat portion. Allow yourself time to deeply relax at the end of your session. You do not have to use all of the following points; using one or two of them when you have a free hand can be effective. Begin by standing with your arms by your sides.

Step 1

Breathing Exercise: Inhale as your arms come up over your head; exhale as they come down. Repeat slowly seven times.

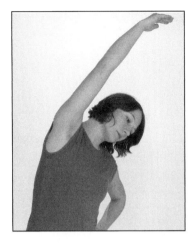

Step 2

Stretch & Self-Massage: Spend three to five minutes slowly stretching tense areas of your body. Breathe deeply into your abdomen and pelvis. Rotate and move your joints, neck, and hips. Take additional time to massage areas that feel tight.

Lie down on your back. Prop a pillow under your knees for comfort.

Step 3

Hold Both K 27: Place your fingertips on both K 27 points (in the hollows below the inside edge of your collarbones). Close your eyes, and do long, slow, deep breathing for two minutes. Consciously focus on the warmth of your hands. Holding these key points harmonizes the healing channels of the body and regulates hormonal function.

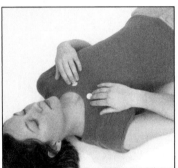

Step 4

Palm CV 17: Place both palms, one over the other, at the center of your breastbone. Breathe into your feelings. Explore the warmth of your own healing energy. Visualize a beautiful summer day as you breathe deeply for two minutes.

Step 5

Hold Sp 12 & Sp 13: Place your fingertips on Sp 12 and Sp 13 (in the middle of the crease where the leg joins the trunk of the body) on both sides. Apply gentle, steady pressure as you breathe deeply into your belly. Take a few minutes to nourish this area lovingly, being grateful for your cycle and for your body's ability to cleanse and renew itself through bleeding.

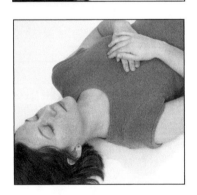

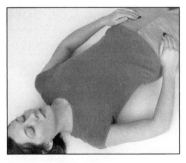

Step 6

Deep Relaxation: Place your hands at your sides, and begin long, slow, deep breathing into your body. Allow ten minutes of relaxation after this powerful acupressure session.

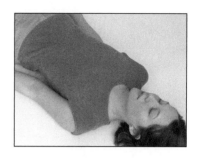

Menstrual Cramps (Dysmenorrhea)

Many women suffer from menstrual cramps. The pain prevents some women from going to work three or more days a month. Lee, a middle-aged professional woman, worked as an advocate for abused women. Every month menstrual cramps incapacitated her completely for four days. Sometimes the pain caused her to throw up. She tried medication and exercise for years with no resolution.

During one of her acupressure sessions, holding points in her pelvic area (CV 6, Sp 12, Sp 13, and B 48) released painful memories of her clients' abuse. The battered women and children in her office felt hopeless. Although Lee tried to not consciously take on her clients' pain, the stories were overwhelming. "I feel like I cramp and bleed for all women," she said. "My body holds the pain and burdens of their world."

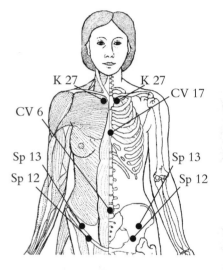

Lee used the following self-care routine to relieve her cramps and pelvic tension. Acupressure unlocked her stored emotional trauma; associated memories surfaced as pressure points were held and her muscular tension melted. She also learned breathing affirmations for releasing the burdens of her clients. After one month of practicing acupressure and daily stretching, her symptoms resolved. As a result, she furthered her preventive skills and went on to teach self-acupressure in her clinic.

Emotional stress and frustration directly affect the pain a woman feels during her cycle. Sexual abuse and trauma, unfulfilling sexual relationships, and the inability to say no often constrict muscles in the pelvic region. Excessive or extreme cramping can also be a signal of a serious imbalance in your body. If cramps become severe or continue, consult your physician and practice this self-care routine daily.

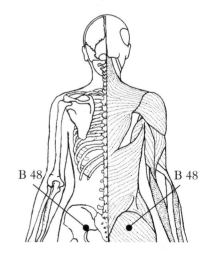

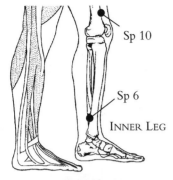

Sp 10

Sp 6

INNER LEG

SELF-CARE ROUTINE FOR
MENSTRUAL CRAMPS

Most of this routine will be done lying on your side. Create a healing environment to deeply relax. Choose a mat, sleeping bag, or bed with pillows and blankets to make yourself comfortable. Begin in a sitting position.

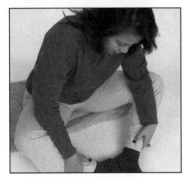

Step 1

Foot Massage: Apply gradual, firm pressure to all areas of your feet as you massage and squeeze them for two minutes. Rotate and pull each toe. Knead and squeeze the ankles, paying particular attention to the Achilles tendon; this area contains acupressure points that relax the uterus. Press along the instep, and hold whatever areas feel tense or sore.

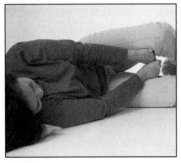

Step 2

Firmly Hold Sp 6: Breathe deeply as you use firm, steady pressure on Sp 6 (four finger-widths above the inside anklebone) for one minute on each side. Encourage your body to unwind by repeating the affirmation "I allow my body to relax and be at peace."

Now lie comfortably on your side.

Step 3

Hold Both Sp 10: Stack your fists, one on top of the other, three finger-widths above the inner kneecap on the inside edge of your legs. As you bring your knees together, the sides of your fists press both Sp 10 points. Allow your right leg to lie on top of your right fist, letting the weight of your legs create the pressure. Close your eyes, and take long, slow, deep breaths for two minutes. Cover yourself with a blanket if you feel chilly. Sp 10 is associated with worry, sweet cravings, cramping, and reproductive imbalances.

Step 4

Palm CV 6: Apply light pressure, two finger-widths below the navel, with one hand over the other. Focus your attention on the warmth of your hands. Close your eyes, and breathe deeply for two minutes. Use your breath to send healing energy into this area of your body.

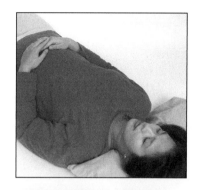

Step 5

Hold CV 17 with GV 26: Place your right fingertip between your upper lip and your nose (GV 26). Place the fingertips of your left hand on the center of your breastbone (CV 17). This combination relieves cramping and relaxes the body. Breathe deeply into your fingertips, affirming deep relaxation for two minutes.

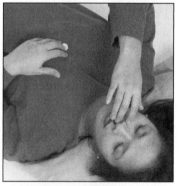

Step 6

Hold H 1: With both hands, reach across to the opposite armpit creases to lightly hold H 1. Breathe deeply into your heart for two minutes to fully benefit from this soothing and relaxing point.

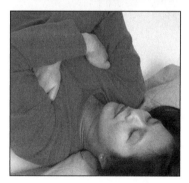

Step 7

Deep Relaxation: Spend five to fifteen minutes lying on your side deeply relaxing. Cover yourself with a blanket to prevent chilling. Close your eyes and fall asleep to deeply nourish your body.

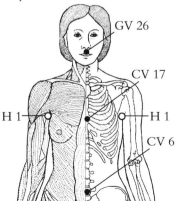

○ – H 1 is in the center of the armpit.

Affirmations for Menopause

• *I listen to the messages of my body with compassion.*

• *I am breathing deeply and accepting how my body is changing.*

• *Menopause is teaching me to surrender to nature and trust myself.*

• *I am learning to love myself more and more through each life passage.*

• *Menopause strengthens my ability to make wise choices in my life.*

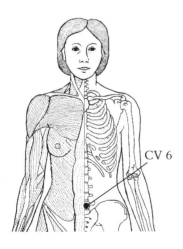

CV 6

Perimenopause & Menopause

Lori, a middle-aged professional woman and mother of four children, described her menopausal symptoms as happening overnight: "I woke up at two A.M. sweating and uncomfortable. My mind was racing. I couldn't get back to sleep for hours. When I woke up in the morning, my skin was crawling and my feelings jumped from one extreme to another. That morning my husband asked if there was an impostor at the breakfast table. I was terrified by my emotions and symptoms. I felt like I was going crazy!"

Acupressure benefits perimenopausal and menopausal imbalances in several ways. Holding acupressure points while breathing deeply releases tension and opens the body's healing energy. There are special acupressure point formulas for relieving mood swings, night sweats, abdominal pain and tension, breast tenderness, heightened emotions, headaches, neck tension, and back pain. In addition, holding the points increases a woman's awareness, acceptance, and compassion for her body. Reducing stress through acupressure can prevent negative emotions and symptoms from forming.

Acceptance of the aging process is a key for emotional balance during perimenopause and menopause. Often women have difficulty with the transition to getting older and the realization of having new limitations. Negative attitudes about aging often result in PMS symptoms during menopause, only without bleeding.

Acupressure is an alternative to drugs and hormone therapy for a variety of perimenopausal and menopausal symptoms. Combining it with other forms of alternative complementary care, such as dietary therapy, herbs, stress reduction, and exercise results in increased effectiveness for managing menopausal imbalances.

In addition to acupressure, we recommend that women consult their physician to discuss individual symptoms and the options of taking calcium, minerals, natural hormone therapy, and other methods. Also explore the risks menopausal women face related to hormone production and osteoporosis due to their lifestyle previous to menopausal years. The amount of bone marrow produced is related to long-term exercise habits. Regular exercise and healthy dietary practices (including the elimination of caffeine and alcohol) can decrease menopausal symptoms.

SELF-CARE ROUTINE FOR
PERIMENOPAUSE & MENOPAUSE

This routine can relieve various discomforts such as hot flashes, bloating, headaches, and mood swings. Practice it sitting in a quiet, private area; wear comfortable clothing.

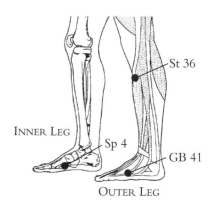

Step 1

Self-Massage & Stretch: Spend five to ten minutes stretching tense areas of your body. Rotate all of your joints, especially your head and shoulders. Breathe deeply as you massage your hands, feet, and neck.

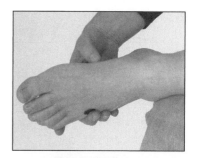

Step 2

Hold Sp 4 with GB 41: Sitting comfortably, firmly grasp hold of Sp 4 (on the arch of your right foot, one finger-width below the ball of the foot) with your thumb and use your fingers to press GB 41 (on the top of the foot, in between the webbing of the fourth and fifth toes). Breathe deeply with your eyes closed for two minutes. Then switch and repeat on the left foot. Holding these points relieves many reproductive and emotional imbalances.

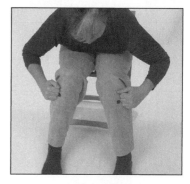

Step 3

Rub St 36: Place your fists over St 36 (four finger-widths below the knee, on the outside of the leg). Using firm friction, rub up and down briskly to stimulate St 36 as you breathe deeply for one minute. Rubbing this point reduces dizziness, fatigue, digestive imbalances, food cravings, mood swings, and worry.

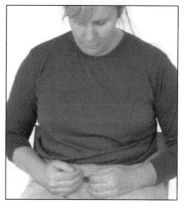

Step 4

Hold CV 6: Use your fingertips to press on CV 6 (two finger-widths below the belly button). Begin long, slow, deep breathing for two minutes to counteract many menopausal challenges.

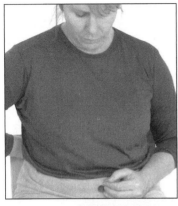

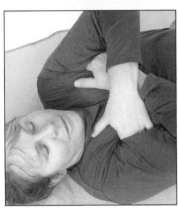

Step 5

Hold CV 6 with GV 4: Continue to keep your left hand on CV 6. Move your right hand to GV 4 (on your back, between the vertebrae at waist level). Breathe deeply as you hold for one minute.

Step 6

Hold Both H 1: Place the fingertips of both hands into the opposite armpit creases (H 1). Breathe deeply, feeling the support of your hands, for one minute. Allow any images, memories, or tears to surface.

Step 7

Relax: Close your eyes, and relax for five minutes. Before getting up, rotate your wrists and ankles, and stretch your body like a cat. Sit up slowly with your spine straight.

Step 8

Press CV 17: Place the palms of your hands together in front of your chest. Allow the knuckles of your thumbs to rest at the center of your breastbone (CV 17). Close your eyes, lower your head, drop your shoulders, and breathe deeply for a minute or two for emotional balancing.

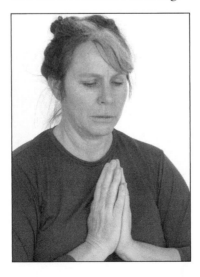

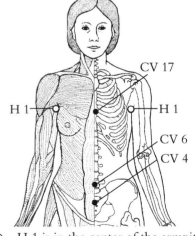

○ – H 1 is in the center of the armpit.

25

NIGHTMARES

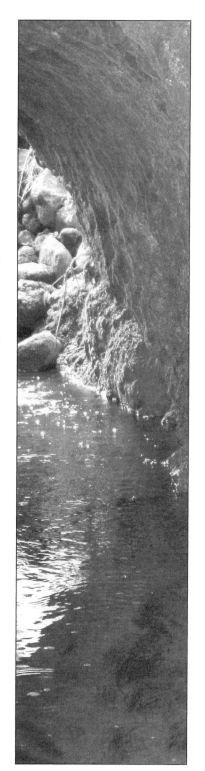

Dreams can reflect your unconscious attitudes and unresolved emotions. They can also provide guidance, nourish your spirit, and enhance your inner awareness. Paying attention to characters and images in your dreams can give you powerful insights. Each character and scene can reflect an intimate part of your self. Such self-awareness contributes to emotional healing and your well-being.

Nightmares can occur for a variety of reasons. During the dream state, our bodymind processes and relives accumulated stress from the day. Illness and high fevers may cause nightmares. Drugs, medications, and poor eating habits, especially before bedtime, can create restless sleep. Nightmares also often follow traumatic events, violent experiences, and loss. Acupressure is effective in treating all of these root causes of nightmares.

Journaling is a powerful way to record and integrate dream messages. Sleep with a notebook near your bedstand so you can record your dreams as soon as you wake up. Drawing and coloring dream stories can tap in to the intuitive wisdom of your inner child. Dreams can give you conscious insight and unleash important details of your subconscious world.

Nick was eight years old when he came to the office with chronic nightmares and migrainelike headache symptoms. His parents believed Nick's headaches were the result of his active imagination. One of his favorite pastimes was watching horror movies on television.

Nick routinely had a big bowl of buttered popcorn and ice cream with his family just before he retired to his own room to watch television. This was a new ritual the family shared in the evening due to a recent change in his father's work schedule; he often wasn't home for dinner. So the children would sit with their dad before bedtime for snacks.

Affirmations to Counteract Nightmares

- *I release any stress and let myself go.*

- *I let myself completely relax; there's nothing in the way of going into a deep sleep.*

- *I am at peace with all my relations.*

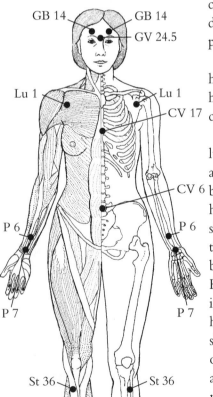

Nick had an acupressure session and he learned points GB 14 and LI 4 for headaches. He also learned a posture for calming himself, which stimulated St 36, Lu 9, P 6, and P 7. His nightmares and headaches stopped a week after he discontinued late-night eating and horror movie watching and practiced the acupressure exercise. Finding relief from headaches and bad dreams was a big enough incentive for him to continue practicing self-acupressure.

Dreams can also reflect the memory of a traumatic experience, as unconscious emotional trauma can release while you are sleeping. But recurring dreams can be unsettling. We recommend the support of a therapist or spiritual counselor to resolve any distressful nightmares that recur.

Shelley had a recurring nightmare when she was twenty-two. It was so provoking that she sought antidepressant and sleep medications. Eventually her physician advised her to consider therapy for resolving her emotional issues since her prescriptions caused nausea, headaches, lethargy, and fatigue. After a year of dream therapy, Shelley was still blocked and unable to make progress. Thus, she began seeking alternative health care.

Shelley was an excellent candidate for acupressure because she had already processed so much with her therapist. Beth guided her into her body and encouraged her to relax while holding the calming points CV 17, P 6, and GV 24.5.

Acupressure deeply relaxed Shelley's body and facilitated a lucid dream state. When she fell asleep, her eyes twitched and anxiety began to build. She felt like a pressure cooker ready to blow. Her breathing sped up. A recurring image of a dark man in her nightmare got closer and closer. Beth held Lu 1 and CV 17 as she coached Shelley to breathe deeply to prevent hyperventilation. Suddenly Shelley's body gripped with pain. Her groin burned, and she felt nauseous, anxious, fearful, and out of control. Holding CV 6 in the lower abdomen released an unforgettable image of her uncle's face. Shelley reexperienced the trauma she had buried since she was four years old. Her body involuntarily shook, releasing the source of her recurring nightmare, the pain of her childhood abuse. Shelley embraced herself in a self-acupressure hug as she cried softly and rocked her body. Her nightmare never recurred after this powerful acupressure session.

Although Shelley was relieved to know the truth behind her nightmare, she was exhausted after her session. She said it took her two weeks to integrate her one-hour session. She continued self-care daily for one month and returned for two more sessions with Beth. She learned shamanic practices to get further closure on her childhood memories. Instead of feeling like a half-person, she felt whole. Acupressure helped Shelley move forward in life without getting stuck in the memory of her buried childhood trauma.

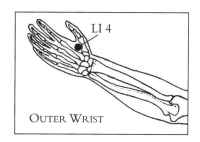

OUTER WRIST

Recovering from a Nightmare

Move into a fetal position on your side. Hug yourself around your knees, and breathe slowly into your heart. This posture is naturally soothing and presses the acupressure points listed below for restoring physical and emotional well-being:

- **St 36** rejuvenates the energy system of the body.

- **Lu 9** restores the spirit through deep breathing.

- **P 6 and P 7** calm traumatic experiences for emotional balancing.

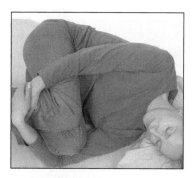

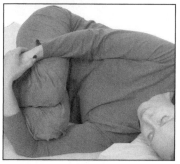

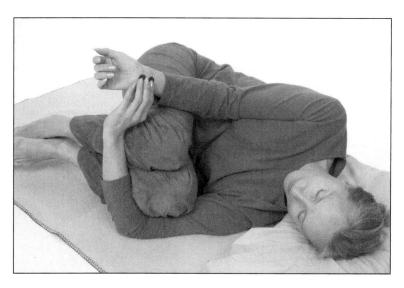

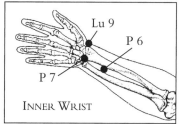

INNER WRIST

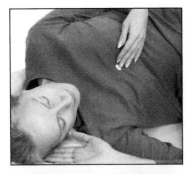

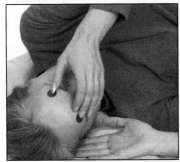

QUICK TIPS FOR NIGHTMARES

Calm Yourself: Immediately after a nightmare, place your fingertips at the center of your breastbone. Holding CV 17 (Sea of Tranquility) can immediately calm you and help relieve the trauma.

Heighten Dream Recall: Lightly touch the GB 14 points in the center of your forehead (a finger-width above your eyebrows). Holding these points can help you recall your dream and release its emotional distress.

SUGGESTIONS FOR ALLEVIATING NIGHTMARES

- **Chamomile Tea** before bed calms the heart and mind.

- **Stretching & Deep Breathing** before bed can relax the body and calm the mind.

- **Foods to Avoid:** alcohol, caffeine, spicy foods, dairy, yeast, and refined sugar products.

- **Foods to Increase:** whole grains rich in calcium such as brown rice, oats, and millet.

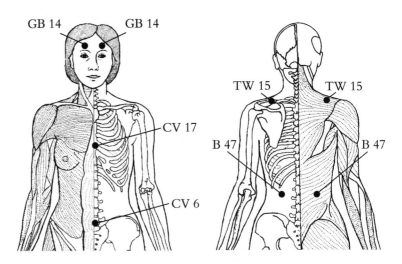

SELF-CARE ROUTINE FOR
NIGHTMARES

Begin this routine with a hot bath, five minutes of stretching, and five minutes of prayer or positive affirmation. Create a healing space with soft lighting and music. Have a blanket nearby for deep relaxation after your session.

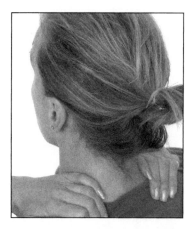

Step 1

Self-Massage: Massage the tightest areas of your body for one to three minutes. Close your eyes and breathe deeply as you enjoy massaging yourself.

Step 2

Hold B 47: Lie down comfortably on your back. Place both hands underneath your lower back, using the knuckles of your fists or your fingertips at waist level to press B 47. Focus on breathing deeply into your lower back for one minute.

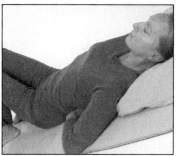

Step 3

Palm CV 6: Bring your hands two finger-widths below the navel, resting your fingertips or palms over CV 6. Apply firm, steady pressure, and breathe deeply into your belly for two minutes. Visualize healing energy circulating up your back and down the front of your body while you affirm the earth's support.

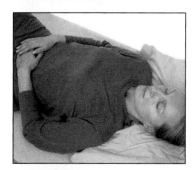

Step 4

Hold TW 15: Reach your hands over the top of your shoulders to grasp the upper edge of the shoulder blade, TW 15. Imagine your body safely within a cocoon of light. Breathe deeply for two minutes as you imagine the warmth of the sun circulating within you.

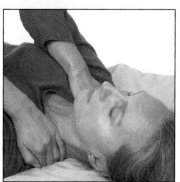

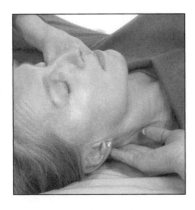

Step 5

Hold GB 20: Glide your fingertips underneath the skull into two hollow spots. Let go of your thoughts and worries. Continue to breathe deeply for two minutes.

Step 6

Final Balancing: Hold GV 20 (at the crown) with GV 24.5 (at the center of the brow) for one minute.

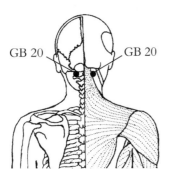

GB 20 — GB 20

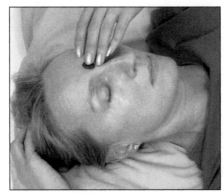

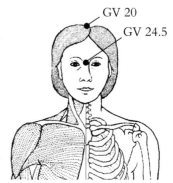

GV 20

GV 24.5

Step 7

Deep Relaxation: Deeply relax for five to fifteen minutes. If you are practicing at night, let yourself go into a deep sleep.

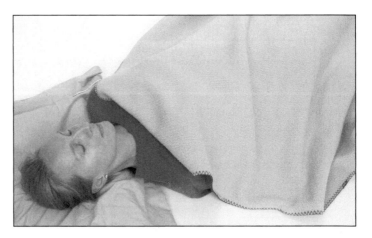

PART IV:

GOING FURTHER

"We find that applying spiritual awareness in daily life is of primary importance and is the one principle most often neglected in regard to food.... Food becomes an ultimate medicine when we recognize it as a facet of our Mind....We recognize both aspects: the spirit teaches about correct diet, and good diet supports spiritual practice....Our goal is that more people begin to follow their inner guidance, in diet and all other areas of their lives."

— Paul Pitchford
Healing with Whole Foods

26

DIET FOR
EMOTIONAL HEALING

This chapter introduces dietary principles and guidelines that can rebuild your body's energy and support emotional healing. Your diet can enhance or hinder acupressure's emotional balancing process; a poor diet can counteract the positive benefits of any therapy. For example, eating mostly raw, cold foods can lower body temperature, tax the digestive system, and produce cold symptoms. Foods containing a high amount of sugar can cause hypoglycemic conditions, mood swings, fatigue, worry, doubt, self-sabotaging patterns, lack of focus, and irritability. Conscious dietary choices, however, optimize acupressure's effectiveness and facilitate personal growth.

Eating wisely is an act of self-love. Loving yourself is essential to receiving universal love and support. When you eat junk foods and feel lousy, you mistreat yourself and are probably making other unhealthy decisions. Making wise food choices supports your health, healing, and spiritual well-being.

Balanced wholesome foods contain natural sources of minerals and vitamins for nourishing your body. When your diet includes adequate nutrients, you are better able to cope with emotional distresses. You can stabilize your emotions and your health by staying away from unhealthy foods and choosing quality foods.

Many foods in the market have very little nutritional value: white flour, soft drinks, and the thousands of highly processed foods with added sugar, corn syrup, oils, salts, and artificial ingredients that contribute to poor health. Fresh fruits, vegetables, and meats have a higher nutritional value. Although preservatives help keep the food on the shelf longer, the added salts and sugars benefit food manufacturers more than consumers.

Healthy attitudes and an awareness of the nutritious properties

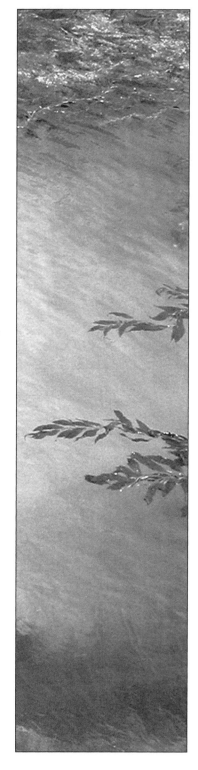

of foods are essential for lifelong change. If you eat foods depleted of vital nutrients (such as processed junk food) for an extended period of time and use minimal variety, your diet can cause an unhealthy condition. Acupressure for emotional stability may be temporary unless you also choose to eat consciously and fortify your body with whole foods.

Cooking for health and vitality is a treasured art. Learn to love and enjoy your food. Whole foods contain natural colors and flavors. They are powerful medicine. Let go of the attitude that a pill, a remedy, or a practitioner will resolve all your problems.

Stress, Diet & Self-Abuse

Pay attention to the food choices you make under stress. Life pressures can trigger emotional issues and challenge our sense of security. Emotional pain coupled with the human desire to be satisfied may cause a person to choose addictive foods high in saturated fats and sugars. These foods are temporarily comforting because their congesting properties quickly numb painful, emotional feelings.

Candidiasis, or the overgrowth of a yeastlike fungus in the body, can be the result of choosing too many yeasted breads, nightshades, pasta, fermented products, alcohol, dairy foods, and sugar. Chinese medicine categorizes candida overgrowth with other cold, damp, depleting conditions. Chronic fatigue, bloating, mental confusion, low immunity, excess worry, anxiety, and depression are common symptoms of candidiasis.

Complicated meals that combine several ingredients from various food groups at one time also stress the digestive tract and create fermentation. Overconsuming rich foods can cause indigestion, flatulence, belching, headache, constipation, insomnia, and nightmares. The "comfort" foods you crave can deplete your vitality and make emotional clearing difficult.

Liz was often depressed, resentful, and stressed out. Her negative feelings knotted her stomach. Her rich diet taxed her digestive tract. After years of worrisome thoughts and complaining about poor relationships, chronic abdominal cramping and nausea developed into irritable bowel syndrome.

Self-acupressure provided Liz with temporary relief of depression and worry. Dietary change became the last step in her recovery. Liz didn't want to give up her comfort foods, but then she learned they were a major cause of her emotional instability. She was encouraged to experiment with her diet to discover the benefits for herself. Eating light soup, salads, wholesome grains, and good-quality protein supported her through stressful times. Cutting out highly sugared, fatty, and salted products was essential for eliminating her negative thought patterns and abdominal tension. Liz still enjoys the foods she once loved on occasion, as a special treat. But she no longer uses food as a response to stress or negative feelings.

Pay attention to your appetite in relationship to your emotions. Unresolved feelings can cause your stomach to crave or reject food. Emptiness or longing for companionship may cause your heart to crave immediate satisfaction. Filling yourself up with food may be how you cope with emotional pain. On the other hand, the shock of death at the end of a significant relationship may inhibit hunger altogether. Lightening your diet can support your emotional need for rest and reflective time. Learn to respect what your body is expressing. The natural rhythm of your emotions can guide you to make wise dietary choices if you will listen to it. Children should be taught this simple lesson as well.

Eating in Harmony with Nature

When you are choosing what to eat, consider the cycles of nature, climatic conditions, and your environment. Since the air temperature around you is colder in the morning, eat a warm, cooked meal such as whole grain cereals or soup. At noon, when the sun warms your body temperature, eat cooler foods like salads and sandwiches with protein to boost your metabolism for the afternoon's activities. In the evening, when your environment is cooling, eat a warm, lighter meal. Try to finish eating three hours before bedtime. Your digestive organs also need to rest when you sleep.

The following chart summarizes our suggestions for balanced diet.

Healthy Foods

- Vegetables and seaweed (30 percent)
- Whole grains (30 percent)
- Dairy, seeds, nuts, and oil (10 percent)
- Beans, tofu, miso soup, fish, chicken, and meat (15 percent)
- Fresh fruits (15 percent)

Foods to Avoid

- Processed foods with sugar
- White flour products
- Salt & red meat (eat less)
- Fried foods & dairy products (eat less)
- Artificial ingredients or preservatives
- Coffee, including decaffeinated (drink less)

Fish, poultry, and small amounts of red meat are medicinal for people with chronic fatigue, emotional sensitivity, physical coldness, and candida. The addition of a few ounces of organic meat without hormones and preservatives can rebuild energy. Problems arise when meat is eaten in excess. Cook meat with ample vegetables, ginger, and occasionally spices to counteract potential eliminatory problems.

If you choose vegetarianism, whole grains with seeds, beans, or a dairy product forms a complete protein based on essential amino acids.★

Many vegetarians do not know how to combine the amino acids in foods properly. Eating incomplete protein from raw vegetables and fruit juices for a long period of time can weaken your system and eventually produce depression and chronic fatigue. Your body needs protein for energy. Replacing meat with cheese does not provide the necessary amino acids required for a complete protein. Become knowledgeable of what your body needs to be healthy, especially if you are responsible for feeding a child.

Three meals per day are not necessary. Some people respond better to several light meals, while others respond to two quality meals.

★See Frances Moore Lappé, *Diet for a Small Planet* (New York, Balantine Books, 1971); or Ellen Buchman Ewald, *Recipes for a Small Planet* (New York, Ballantine Books, 1973).

Learn to follow your own natural rhythm as to when to eat, what to eat, and how much is necessary for your body's essential needs.

Before eating, close your eyes and take a moment to breathe deeply and appreciate your food. Appreciate the cycles of nature and the human efforts that went into cultivating the food on your table. The spiritual practice of giving thanks before eating adds to the enjoyment of its flavor and texture.

Eating when you are angry, worried, or upset is counterproductive and can cause digestive problems. Food literally stuffs these feelings down. Instead, breathe deeply, go for a walk, or simply stretch your body. Explore the acupressure routines in this chapter to benefit digestion and release of muscular tension.

Daily Food Guidelines

Check your local bookstore for recipe books for cooking with whole foods. Learning to prepare foods properly is a great investment in your health. The following dietary suggestions can enhance your emotional well-being:

Foods & Substances to Avoid: preservatives, white flour, white and brown sugar, junk food, sodas, caffeine, alcohol, recreational drugs, and tobacco.

Whole Grains: Whole grains reflect the complete life cycle of plants and should comprise at least 30 percent of a balanced daily diet. Their carbohydrate content makes them an excellent energy source. Grains such as brown rice, barley, millet, oats, whole wheat, rye, and corn contain a rich supply of proteins and minerals. Choose organic whole grain flour products instead of those containing bleached or unbleached white flour.

Buckwheat: Classified as an herb seed, buckwheat is excellent for people who need additional body warmth. It is very warming and therefore is a great nutritious food for people who live in colder climates.

Vegetables: Vegetables should comprise at least 30 percent of a balanced diet. They supply important nutrients and support your body's eliminatory functions. Eat vegetables lightly steamed when you are dealing with emotional healing issues. Lightly cooked vegetables aid digestion and facilitate the absorption of essential nutrients. Eating vegetables local to your geographical area adjusts your blood to seasonal changes.

Nightshades: Tomatoes, potatoes, sweet peppers, and eggplants can cause allergies and aggravate arthritic symptoms. Swelling, joint pain, lethargy, and depression are common allergic reactions to the nightshade family. Minimize your use of these foods, especially during times of emotional stress.

Seaweeds: Seaweeds are the most nutritious vegetables due to their high mineral content. Explore using different kinds of seaweeds, such as wakame, hijiki, dulse, and kelp by adding bits of dried seaweed to your soup. Children often find toasted wakame strips delicious to snack on alone or crushed and mixed with popcorn.

Fish, Poultry & Meat: Fish and poultry can strengthen your body's condition. Two to four ounces of organic meat per day, without hormones or preservatives, can rebuild your energy. Too much meat in your diet can cause problems in the digestive tract. Use ginger, garlic, and onions during the cooking process to neutralize bacteria and toxic side effects. In traditional Chinese medicine, certain meats are known to benefit specific organs. Including meat in your diet can relieve many emotional complaints, especially when accompanied by depression and tiredness.

Beans, Seeds & Legumes: These foods should comprise 10 percent of a balanced vegetarian diet. Included within this category are tofu, tempeh, and other soybean products. Beans complement essential amino acids and make a full protein when eaten with grains. Combining foods properly ensures that your body will receive important nutrients. Beans include garbanzos, lentils, peas, black beans, green mungs, aduki, and others. A pressure cooker works well for cooking dried beans at home. Soak for four to eight hours, and add a clove of garlic, one whole onion, and a piece of seaweed or ginger to help relieve gas. Skim off the blackish residue of the beans after they are halfway cooked. Eating an average bowl of rice with a quarter-cup of beans is a balanced ratio for properly combining the amino acids for a full protein. Be sure to eat beans in small quantities since they are a highly concentrated food.

Dairy & Nuts: These foods belong within the 10 percent range of your daily diet. In excess these foods can cause mucus, sluggishness, depression, and congestion, eventually resulting in tumors and lumps. The high oil and fat content of nuts and dairy foods can make digestion difficult. Gulping milk or eating large slabs of cold cheese can cause digestive problems. Warming dairy products can make them more digestible. Yogurt adds healthy bacteria to your system. Milk alternatives include soymilk, rice milk, and nut milk. Nut butters from almonds, cashews, sunflowers, or peanuts can also provide healthy alternatives to cheese.

Fats & Oils: These foods belong within the 5 to 10 percent range of your daily diet. Despite dietary fads, completely eliminating fat and oil is not healthful. These foods are essential for providing internal heat, protecting the internal organs, and synthesizing fat-soluble vitamins. Virgin olive oil, sesame oil, and flaxseed oil are the healthiest choices. Proper storage is essential for these foods to retain their nutritional value. Fats and oils easily turn rancid from exposure to light and air. Transfer store-bought oils from plastic to glass containers, and store them in the refrigerator under cool, unlit conditions.

Fruits: These foods should comprise 10 to 15 percent of a balanced diet, depending upon the season. They are cleansing and assist in eliminating waste materials in the digestive tract. Excessive fruit or fasting can overcleanse and damage your digestive and circulatory systems. Fruit is digested more easily if you live in a warm climate. Eating excess fruit in the winter can cause metabolic problems, mood swings, depression, and other emotional imbalances. Mixing half fruit juice and half mineral or spring water is a good alternative to sugared soda products.

Healthy Snacks: Vegetable sticks, raisins, nuts (like almonds), and organic apples are healthy choices.

Beverages: A simple glass of water with a squeeze of lemon in the morning can be cleansing. This natural drink can also relieve excessive anger.

Meal Suggestions

These suggestions are not intended to constitute a strict regimen.

Morning

- Hot cereal, miso soup, or congee★, with whole grain toast
- Rice or other grains with vegetables and two ounces of protein

Noon

- Healthy sandwich on whole grain bread
- Light soup or broth
- Vegetable sticks
- Whole grain cookie

Evening

- Three ounces of fish
- Steamed vegetables
- Mixed green salad
- Baked yam
- Half-cup brown rice

Drinking with Meals

Gulping fluids while eating can dilute essential digestive enzymes. Try to drink thirty minutes before or after a meal. A light soup or broth during a meal will not hamper digestion; they contain beneficial nutrients and enzymes.

Iced drinks can temporarily paralyze the stomach and impair the digestive system. Avoid iced products entirely during cold and damp seasons. If you do choose to drink a warming fluid with meals, there are numerous herbal teas to select from. Choose a decaffeinated herbal tea such as mint, chamomile, or green tea. Hot water with lemon and grain drinks are excellent alternatives to coffee.

Food Combining

Each food group requires different enzymes and amounts of time to be thoroughly digested. Fermentation and putrefaction occur when incompatible food groups are eaten together. As you become more conscious of proper food combining and experience the properties of healthy foods, your diet will become a storehouse of nutrients and vitality. The following lists show compatible and incompatible food combinations as well as common causes of indigestion.

Food Combinations to Avoid

- Fruits with vegetables
- Fruits with proteins
- Proteins of different varieties together

Foods to Combine

- Vegetables with starches
- Vegetables with proteins
- Fruits with other fruits (except melons)
- Fats and oils with vegetables
- Acidic fruits with proteins or fats

Causes of Indigestion

- Emotional stress
- Overeating
- Overuse of processed, devitalized food
- Foods high in fat, dairy, and sugar
- Improper food combinations
- Abdominal stress and tension
- Lack of daily exercise and stretching
- Eating too much spicy food

★Recipe for congee appears on pages 269–270.

ACUPRESSURE POINTS FOR BALANCING
APPETITE & DIGESTION

From the following list, select one or two key points related to digestion. Hold for two to three minutes. Refer to Part II for acupressure points related to specific conditions.

LI 4, Hoku (located in the webbing between the thumb and index finger, at the highest spot of the muscle that protrudes when the thumb and index finger are brought close together): Holding LI 4 detoxifies the body and relieves allergies, constipation, and sinus pain.

GV 26, Center of the Person (located two-thirds of the way between the upper lip and the nose): Holding GV 26 clears the mind, curbs the appetite, and relieves allergies, pain, and dizziness.

Sp 16, Abdominal Sorrow (located below the edge of the ribcage, a half-inch in from the nipple line): Holding Sp 16 relieves emotional upset and diaphragmatic tension and balances appetite and food cravings.

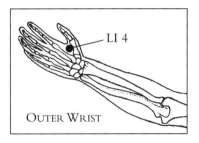

OUTER WRIST

Sp 10, Sea of Blood (located on the inner thigh, four finger-widths above the kneecap): Holding Sp 10 balances mood swings, relieves sugar cravings, and helps regulate the menstrual cycle.

St 36, Three Mile (located four finger-widths below the outside kneecap, one finger-width outside the shinbone): Holding St 36 relieves mood swings, fatigue, indigestion, and nausea; it also reinforces emotional stability, tones the muscles, and aids digestion.

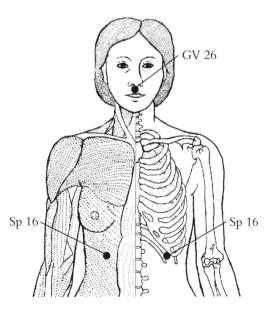

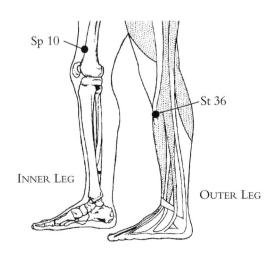

SELF-ACUPRESSURE FOR
DIETARY CHANGE

Emotional imbalances can be aggravated by poor food choices. The following self-care routine can help your body eliminate toxins during dietary change. Gentle stretching, acupressure massage, and point holding are combined to rebalance circulation in the meridian pathways. Practice this routine on an empty stomach or two to four hours after eating a heavy meal.

Begin in a standing position. Have a mat or pad available for comfort during the floor portion of the exercise.

Step 1

Hip Rotations: Stand comfortably with your feet a shoulder-width apart. Rotate your hips slowly in each direction for one minute. Breathe deeply, and focus your attention on the movement of your body. Take a moment to massage your shoulders and neck.

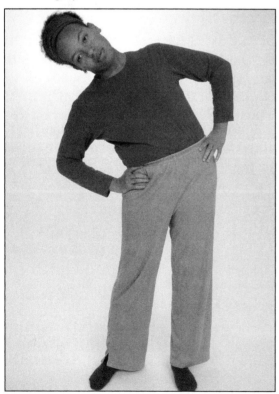

Now lie down comfortably on your back with your knees bent, feet flat on the floor. Remember to breathe deeply during steps 2 to 4 of this routine.

Step 2

Press Elbow Points: Using your thumb, press LI 11 (at the end of the elbow crease at the joint). Firmly press this point for one minute as you rock your knees gently from side to side. Switch and repeat this exercise, holding the LI 11 point on your other arm for one minute.

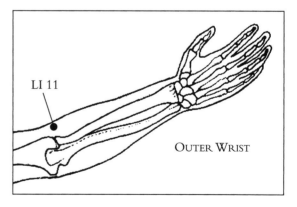

LI 11

OUTER WRIST

Step 3

Abdominal Massage: Move your hands to the top of your abdomen. Using all your fingertips, slowly massage in a clockwise direction. Cover an area about the size of your palm. Repeat for three complete circles. Then completely relax your legs on the floor, and palm your belly for one minute.

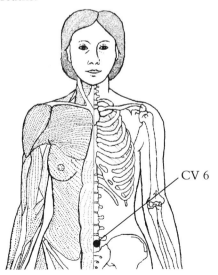

Step 4

Firmly Press CV 6: Place all your fingertips two inches directly below your belly button. Press firmly for one minute as you take long, deep breaths.

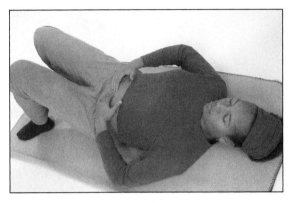

Step 5

Briskly Rub St 36: Place your left heel on your right St 36 point (four finger-widths below the kneecap, toward the outside of the shinbone). If you are on the correct spot, a muscle should pop out when you flex your foot up and down. Briskly rub for one minute, then switch to the other leg. Holding St 36 revitalizes the body and strengthens the digestive system.

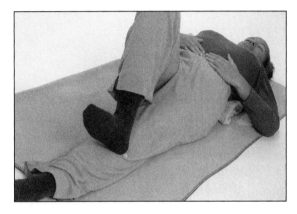

Step 6

Deeply Relax: After stimulating the acupressure points in this exercise, take five to fifteen minutes to close your eyes and relax. Cover yourself with a blanket to avoid getting chilled.

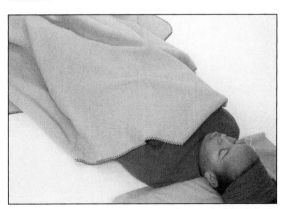

MINIROUTINE FOR COUNTERACTING
FALSE HUNGER

Hunger pains may reflect the need to fill an emotional void. For best results, practice this self-care miniroutine twice a day. If you are still hungry afterward, choose healthy whole foods. Deep breathing during self-acupressure increases circulation, washes away tension, and fills your body with natural vitality.

Begin by placing a towel roll underneath your lower back at waist level. This will stimulate the overall body-strengthening points B 23 and B 47 (two to four finger-widths out from the spine). Keep the towel roll in position during the full routine. Do not use the towel roll if you suffer from disintegrating disks, or broken or fractured bones.

Step 1

Firmly Hold Both St 3: Using your index fingers, lightly press upward into the slight hollow underneath each cheekbone, directly in line with the pupils of the eyes, for one minute. Breathe deeply as you explore this area of your body. Consciously holding these points over a period of two months helped several of our clients stop habitual overeating. Overeating is a common way to stuff, avoid, and numb painful feelings. Tension in the mouth and jaw can be caused by emotional pain, by not being heard or able to express yourself.

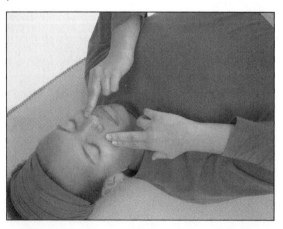

Step 2

Lightly Press Both St 16: Place both middle fingers just above each breast, in line with the nipple. Feel for a sore, tender spot (St 16) in an indentation between the ribs. Hold these points for two minutes as you breathe deeply. Holding St 16 nourishes the emotions and clears melancholy and depression. Using St 16 along with meditation, affirmation, and visualization can curb an emotional appetite and replace a broken heart with self-loving thoughts and feelings.

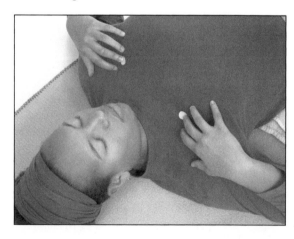

Step 3

Hold Center of Belly (CV 12): Hold this point, located on the midline of the body, three finger-widths below the base of the breastbone, in the pit of the upper stomach.★ As you breathe consciously into your belly for two minutes, ask yourself what you really need in your life. Are you hungry for food, or does your hunger reflect deeper feelings?

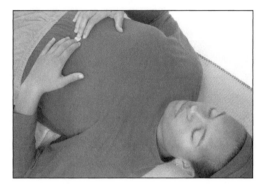

Step 4

Firmly Hold GV 26 with CV 6: Using your right hand, place the tip of your index finger on GV 26 (two-thirds of the way up from the upper lip to the nose). Place the fingertips of your left hand on CV 6 (two finger-widths below the navel), pressing firmly. Breathe deeply into this point combination to balance and stabilize food cravings.

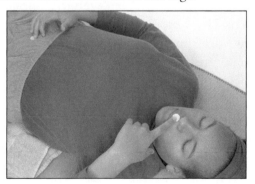

Step 5

Lightly Touch the Third Eye with GV 20: Place the tip of your right middle finger lightly on the Third Eye point, GV 24.5 (between your eyebrows). Use your left fingertips to hold GV 20 (on the crown of your head). To find the Hundred Meeting point (GV 20), draw a line from the back of your ears to the top of your head. Close your eyes, and take long, slow, deep breaths to calm and nourish yourself.

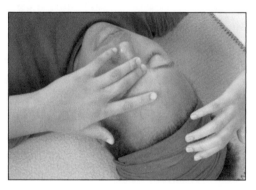

Step 6

Deeply Relax. Let your hands float down to relax at your sides. Close your eyes, and feel the vitality from your breath circulating throughout your body. Focus on your conviction to heal yourself. Continue to relax deeply for five to fifteen minutes.

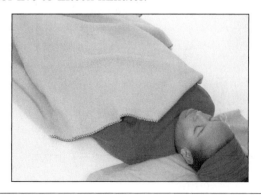

★Do not hold this point deeply if you have a serious medical illness or have just eaten.

RECIPES FOR LIGHT EATING

During times of emotional stress and tension, you may not feel hungry, yet your body still needs essential nutrients and calories to function. Consider these simple food recipes to be medicinal for your body. Explore and experiment with each one, and alter them according to your own tastes and preferences.

Nutritious Broths & Soups

Vegetable broths and healthy bouillon are easy to digest for light eating; your health food store should carry several varieties. Although normally eaten at lunch or dinnertime, soup can be an ideal food for the morning meal. The liquid content rehydrates the body after sleep and, depending on the ingredients, alkalizes the body. Soup or broth can also be a good way to break a fast. Light broths can quickly reduce or eliminate headache and indigestion, especially when associated with emotional distress, overuse of sugar, or excessive environmental stress. Use clear broths for expelling toxins when eliminatory and digestive functions are taxed.

Miso Soup

Miso is a fermented soybean paste made from grains, soybeans, and sea salt. It is a good source of protein, vitamin B, and friendly bacterial enzymes. (All fermented products, including miso, can be contraindicated for yeast allergies, candida, and salt restrictions. If you have any of these conditions, consult a health care provider.) Try this delicious miso soup as a breakfast food or light evening meal.

1 ft. strip of wakame or other seaweed
1 tbsp. sesame oil
1 large onion, chopped
1 c. sliced carrot
2 celery stalks
3 c. water
1 c. sliced chard or kale
½ c. fresh chives or green onion
2 tbsp. miso paste

Miso Soup Option

Add ½ c. cooked beans, cubed fresh tofu, or other protein food for more substance.

Directions:
1. Presoak seaweed and cut into strips.
2. Heat sesame oil in a large pot, and sauté onion, then the carrot, and celery. Remove from heat.
3. In another kettle boil the water; reduce heat to simmer. Add the sautéd vegetables and seaweed to simmer for 10 minutes.
4. Add the chard and chives; cook an additional 5 minutes. Remove pan from heat.
5. Add miso paste into the soup, without heating the miso and thereby killing its valuable digestive enzymes. First remove one half-cup of the broth, stir in the miso paste until it mixes into the broth, and then mix this into the soup.
6. Cover soup and allow to sit for 2 to 5 minutes. Serves 4.

Benefits: Miso soup aids digestion, warms the body, and can decrease feelings of worry, emotional instability, emotional overwhelm, and the inability to focus.

Ginger & Squash Soup

This delicious, nutritious squash soup is colorful and easy to prepare.

1 large or 2 medium carrots, chopped
1 medium onion, chopped
1 large ginger root (4 in.), grated
5 tsp. organic unrefined oil
1 squash (acorn, butternut, or buttercup), peeled and cubed
6-inch strip of kombu (a form of seaweed, available at your health food store)
7 c. water, as needed
Herbal seasoning, to taste: dulse flakes, fresh parsley (chopped), or chives (chopped)

Directions:
1. Sauté carrots, onion, and ginger in oil. Add squash, kombu, and enough water to cover the ingredients.
2. Simmer for 20–30 minutes. Remove from heat.
3. Puree in a blender, adjusting the liquid for desired creaminess. Add seasoning, return to heat, and simmer 5–10 more minutes.
4. Serve garnished with dulse flakes, fresh parsley, or chopped chives.

Congee (Shi Zhou)

Congee is a whole grain cereal diluted to a porridge consistency. Additional beans or animal protein, Chinese herbs, and vegetables are added for therapeutic health reasons. Congee has been used for centuries in Asia for patients with weak digestive systems and mental/emotional instabilities.

To prepare congee, you will need a slow cooker or Crock-Pot. Congee must cook for a long period of time over slow heat. You can prepare this simple food in the evening before bedtime and in the morning wake up to a nourishing breakfast porridge. Congee makes a delicious simple meal for times when stress or indigestion reduces your appetite. It can be divided into individual servings, refrigerated, and eaten consecutively over a number of days. For best results, experiment with each type of congee three days in a row.

Congee Rebuilding Recipe

1 c. organic short-grain brown rice
7 c. water
½ c. wheat gluten or mung beans (substitute organic chickpeas or adzuki beans)
⅛ c. grated ginger (substitute ⅛ c. grated radish if ginger is too spicy)
½ c. water chestnuts (optional)
½ c. fresh burdock root (available at health food store or Asian market)
2 umeboshi plums (available at health food store or Asian herb store)
½ c. organic dandelion or other dark greens, finely chopped (as a garnish)

Directions:
1. Place the rice and water in a slow cooker before bedtime. Add additional ingredients except dandelion or other greens, and stir gently into the pot.
2. Cook overnight about eight hours, until porridge consistency.
3. Garnish with greens as desired for a delicious breakfast porridge. Serves three or four.

Benefits: Rebuilds energy; counteracts depression, grief, numbness, lowered libido, and fatigue. The Congee Rebuilding Recipe contains proteins, spices, and roots that increase body heat and emotional stability.

Congee Calming Recipe

1 c. organic millet
7 c. water
½ c. Chinese yam (or organic yam)
½ c. Jujube dates (or 2 bread dates, chopped)
½ c. chopped celery
1 piece dried wakame, soaked and pre-cut

Directions:

1. Heat the millet and water in a slow cooker for 30 minutes.

2. Then add the other ingredients, stirring gently.

3. Cook overnight, or about eight hours until porridge consistency. Serves three or four.

Benefits: This calming recipe is good for relieving nervousness, decreasing body heat, and reducing tension. Emotionally, this dish counteracts anger, frustration, self-abuse, anxiety, and insomnia. The combination of sweeter grains, yam, and jujube dates calms the body.

Self-Care Routine for
Dietary Change

The following routine can enhance your body awareness and support beneficial changes in your diet through holding two key points. Holding the first point, on the abdomen (CV 6), increases your awareness of your intestines. Feeling your lower abdominal area can motivate you to improve your diet and exercise more. Holding the second point, between the eyebrows (GV 24.5), can help you envision transformational dietary vows.

Take a moment before eating to collect yourself. Place your palms together at the center of the breastbone, so your thumb knuckles press CV 17. Close your eyes and breathe deeply, being thankful for the nourishment the earth provides. Practice this routine daily for best results.

Step 1

Hold CV 6 (Sea of Energy): Hold this point (located three finger-widths below your belly button, in your lower abdomen) with all your fingertips. Curve your fingers, and apply firm pressure gradually in toward your lower spine. Breathe deeply into your stomach with your eyes closed. Ask yourself what your body needs. Continue to breathe deeply into your intestines as you affirm what dietary changes you want to make. Continue for two or three minutes as you say to yourself, "I digest experiences in my life easily."

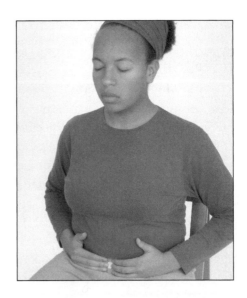

Step 2

Touch GV 24.5 (Third Eye): Close your eyes, and bring your palms together. Use your middle and index fingers to lightly touch the Third Eye point, between your eyebrows. Close your eyes and take long, slow, deep breaths as you envision eating to nourish and heal your body. Bring this intent to your Third Eye point as you continue to breathe deeply for two minutes.

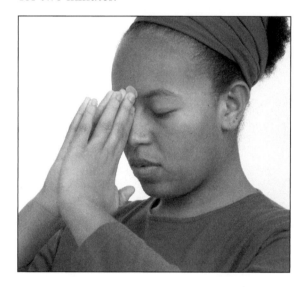

Throughout the process of purification, the individual can be expected to have a number of healing reactions from the residues of past experiences. The cells of the body—in particular those of the brain and liver—are actively encoded with every emotional or mental issue that has not been resolved.

— Paul Pitchford
Healing with Whole Foods

Step 3

Relax: Finish this routine by letting your hands float down into your lap. Feel the vitality from your breath circulating throughout your body. Keep your spine straight, and meditate on your intention to heal yourself.

Learn to trust your feelings and body awareness as your primary guide for choosing the foods that are truly good for you and feel right to your body. The more you follow your "gut feelings," the wiser your choices will become.

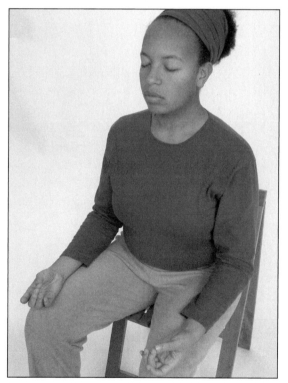

Appendix A:

Top Acupressure Points for Emotional Healing

——————— Facial Points ———————

Point #	Point Name	Point Location	Point Function	Physical Imbalances	Emotional & Spiritual Aspects
GV 24.5	*Third Eye*	Between the eyebrows, in the indentation where the bridge of the nose meets the forehead	Balances the function of the pituitary gland; dispels wind and clears heat; opens the nose	Relieves hay fever, sinus pain, headache, hot flashes, dizziness, hypertension, insomnia, eye irritation	Spiritual and emotional healing point; calms the spirit; relieves anxiety, depression, anger; heals trauma
GB 14	*Clear Mind*	On the forehead, one finger-width above the eyebrows, in line with the pupil	Brightens and clears the eyes; dispels wind, heat, and cold; clears the mind	Relieves eyestrain, head congestion, mental stress, headache, eye twitch, sore eyes	Emotional balancing point; relieves anger, irritability, anxiety, panic attacks, worry, trauma, addiction
St 6	*Jaw Chariot*	On the jaw muscle (masseter), between the upper and lower jaw	Relaxes the jaw muscle; moistens the throat; dispels wind, cold, and heat	Relieves TMJ pain, jaw inflammation, jaw pain, grinding teeth, mumps, neck stiffness, and toothache	Heals childhood emotional trauma; relieves chronic worry, self-abuse, phobia, terror, resentment, addiction
St 3	*Facial Beauty*	Under the cheekbone, directly down from the pupil	Opens the eyes and sinuses; relaxes the facial muscles; governs facial circulation	Relieves stuffy nose, sinus congestion, eye irritation, headache, toothache, facial pain, facial paralysis, nausea	Clears the mind; relieves self-doubt, spiritual stagnation; opens the windows of the sky points

Point #	Point Name	Point Location	Point Function	Physical Imbalances	Emotional & Spiritual Aspects
GV 26	*Center of the Person*	On the midline between the base of the nose and the top of the upper lip	Clears the brain and the nose; alleviates pain; dispels wind and heat	Relieves cramps, fainting, dizziness, hay fever, eye muscle twitches and cramps, lower back pain, spasms, and stiffness	Revives consciousness and morale; calms and restores the spirit after trauma; relieves depression with uncontrolled weeping
CV 24	*Supporting Nourishment*	Midway between the center of the lower lip and chin	Transforms cold, wind, heat, dampness, phlegm	Relieves facial tension, lockjaw, voice loss, throat spasm, tightness	Releases emotional pain and trauma; opens vulnerability; relieves emotional numbness

——— NECK, SHOULDER & BACK POINTS ———

Point #	Point Name	Point Location	Point Function	Physical Imbalances	Emotional & Spiritual Aspects
GB 21	*Shoulder Well*	On the top of the shoulder muscle, one inch out from the base of the lower neck	Benefits the shoulder area; softens hard masses; facilitates lactation; expedites labor	Relieves fatigue, shoulder tension, stiff neck, nervous problems, poor circulation	Releases burdens, uptightness, grief, depression, anxiety, nervousness, fear, self-abuse, addiction, jealousy, and codependency
B 15 B 36– B 38	*Vital Diaphragm* *Emotional Support*	Between the shoulder blades and the spine, at the level of the heart	Regulates and benefits the respiratory and cardiovascular systems; relieves upper body pain	Relieves breathing difficulty, anxiety, hypertension; calms the emotions and promotes relaxation	Calms the spirit for spiritual renewal; emotional healing point for regaining spirit after trauma
SI 10	*Shoulder Blade Concerns*	In the joint where the back of the arm meets the back; in the hollow formed by the scapulohumeral articulation	Regulates circulation into the arm and hand; regulates blood pressure; relieves pain in the shoulder blade and arm	Upper back or shoulder pain, stiff neck, arm problems (pain, tingling, numbness, poor circulation, cold hands), hypertension, insomnia	Spiritual unrest; stuck in sadness, shame, guilt, jealousy, anger, resentment, abuse, depression, addictive behavior, codependency; good for enhancing creativity

Point #	Point Name	Point Location	Point Function	Physical Imbalances	Emotional & Spiritual Aspects
TW 15	*Heavenly Rejuvenation*	In the shoulders, midway from the base of neck to the outside of the shoulders, one inch below the top of the shoulders	Relaxes shoulder muscles; dispels wind and cold; balances body temperature; builds resistance to colds and flu	Relieves shoulder pain, exhaustion, fatigue, poor circulation, stiff neck, nervousness, chronic fatigue, lung and skin problems	Governs emotional adaptability; relieves resentment, self-abuse, anger, jealousy, fear, codependency, anxiety
GV 16	*Wind Mansion*	In the center of the back of the head, in the large hollow under the base of the skull	Clears the head and the nose; opens the sensory organs; dispels wind	Relieves neck pain, headache, sore throat, dizziness, hypertension, cold, insomnia	Root of the spirit world; promotes clearheadedness; relieves trauma and shock, nightmares, fear, terror, numbness
B 10	*Heavenly Pillar*	One thumb-width below the base of the skull, on the ropy muscles a half-inch out from the spine	Opens the sensory organs; relaxes the body; calms the nerves	Relieves insomnia, burnout, stress, over-exhaustion, stiff neck, sore throat, eyestrain, heaviness in the head, thyroid imbalance	Pillar of spirit; relieves anxiety, emotional distress, depression, fear, phobia, self-abuse, addictive behavior, codependency
GB 20	*Gates of Consciousness*	In the hollow below the base of the skull, three finger-widths out from the midline	Governs relaxation and circulation through the brain; brightens the eyes, clears the senses	Relieves headache, hypertension, stiff neck, uptightness, general pain, insomnia, eyestrain, dizziness, and head cold	Heals traumatic experiences; heightens spirituality; balances jealousy, resentment, irritability, addiction, guilt, numbness, anger, and judgment

FRONTAL POINTS

Point #	Point Name	Point Location	Point Function	Physical Imbalances	Emotional & Spiritual Aspects
Sp 12 Sp 13	*Rushing Door* *Mansion Cottage*	In the middle of the crease where the leg joins the trunk of the body	Governs circulation through the abdomen; facilitates mind-body balance; transforms damp heat	Relieves menstrual cramps, abdominal pain and discomfort, edema, reproductive problems, hernia, endometriosis	Relieves frustration, irritability, guilt, phobia, shame, emotional numbness, self-abuse, worry, mood swings
St 36	*Three Mile*	On the outside of the leg, four finger-widths below the bottom of the kneecap	Strengthens the stomach, spleen, kidney, and lung; balances digestion and appetite; benefits the knees; tones the muscles	Relieves exhaustion, chronic fatigue, upset stomach, indigestion, nausea, constipation, muscular problems, knee pain; restores the immune system	Wellness point; relieves anxiety, panic attacks, mood swings, abandonment issues, depression, self-abuse and self-esteem issues, worry, codependency
Sp 16	*Abdominal Sorrow*	Below the edge of the ribcage, at the junction of the eighth and ninth rib cartilage, just medial to the nipple line	Governs digestion and appetite disorders; regulates circulation though the diaphragm	Indigestion, belching, side aches, diaphragm tension, hiccups, snoring, insomnia, liver and gall bladder disorders	Balances poor image, esteem problems, feelings of powerlessness, chronic worry, guilt, sorrow, grief, codependency, and abandonment issues
Lv 3 GB 41	*Happy Calm* *Above Tears*	On the top of the foot, in the valley between the bones of second and large toe (Lv 3); the fourth and fifth toe (GB 41)	Alleviates congestion; regulates the liver and gall bladder; alleviates pain	Relieves arthritis, cramps, headaches, tired painful eyes, insomnia, abdominal distention, shoulder pain, hypertension	Soul healing point; relieves irritability; balances resentment, jealousy, anger, attitude problems, judgment

—————— Chest Points ——————

Point #	Point Name	Point Location	Point Function	Physical Imbalances	Emotional & Spiritual Aspects
CV 17	*Sea of Tranquility*	On the center of the breastbone, four finger-widths up from the base of the breastbone, in an indentation	Calms and relaxes the body; releases the chest; regulates cardiovascular functions and nourishes the heart	Nervousness, difficult breathing, chest tension or congestion, insufficient lactation, heart palpitations, chest pain, dizziness, anxiety	Emotional balancing; relieves depression, grief, sadness, anguish, emotional trauma; balances the emotions and calms the spirit
St 12 St 13 St 16	*Broken Bowl* *Chi Door* *Breast Window*	Above and below the middle of the collarbone Above the breast tissue, in line with the nipples	Regulates energy flow through the throat and chest; governs the breast tissue and lactation; regulates and relaxes chest muscles	Relieves chest tension, pain, and soreness, cough, asthma, bronchitis, breast pain, lactation, breathing problems, heartburn, insomnia	Supports emotional openness and healing; relieves depression, melancholia, grief, sadness, trauma, emotional distress
K 27 K 24– K 26	*Elegant Mansion* *Spirit Storage*	In the hollow directly below the protrusions of the collarbone and each of the rib spaces below	Expands and relaxes chest; benefits the kidneys, lungs, and stomach	Relieves breathing difficulties, asthma, sore throat, coughing, thyroid problems	Gathers and opens the spirit; relieves panic, fear, anxiety, grief, emotional exhaustion, and disorientation
Lu 1	*Letting Go*	On the upper outer portion of the chest, three finger-widths below the collarbone	Benefits the lungs; clears chest congestion and repressed emotions	Relieves breathing problems, coughing, asthma, chest tension, congestion, or pain, skin disorders	Opens the spirit; releases anxiety, emotional holding, expectations, depression, grief, sadness, and anger

ARMS & ABDOMEN POINTS

Point #	Point Name	Point Location	Point Function	Physical Imbalances	Emotional & Spiritual Aspects
H 7	*Spirit Gate*	On the little finger side of the forearm at the crease of the wrist, in the depression of the protruding bone	Clears and regulates the heart; benefits the tongue; clears the brain	Relieves insomnia, distress, anxiety, dizziness, insanity, delirious speech, forgetfulness, disorientation, urinary incontinence, headache, impotence	Calms the spirit; treats spiritual disorders such as chronic distress, annoyance, mania, poor memory, depression, insomnia; relieves sadness, anxiety
P 6	*Inner Gate*	P 6: Three finger-widths above center of inner wrist crease	Calms the internal organs; regulates the heart, liver, and stomach; benefits the diaphragm	Relieves nausea, upset stomach, morning sickness, indigestion, epilepsy, carpal tunnel, wrist tendinitis pain, insomnia, dizziness	Emotional balancing, spiritual calming point; relieves anger, anxiety, nervousness, panic attack, fear, phobia, addiction, mood swings
P 7	*Big Mound*	P 7: Center of inner wrist crease			
P 8	*Labor Palace*	P 8: Center of palm			
P 9	*Balanced Love*	Tip of the third finger, at the base of the nail	Revives consciousness; clears heat	Relieves shock, coma, convulsion, chest or gastric pain, hot palms	Calms the spirit; relieves resentment, anger, frustration, irritability, anxiety, sadness, remorse
CV 4	*First Gate*	Two, three, and four finger-widths below the navel on the midline of the lower abdomen	Revives the body's healing processes; benefits the kidneys; develops and restores vitality; strengthens the waterways and the reproductive system	Relieves stomachache, abdominal mass, menstrual cramping, insomnia, urinary incontinence, impotence, infertility, chronic fatigue, constipation, headache	Good for developing emotional stability and deepening spiritual awareness; strengthens sense of self; used for self-abuse, addiction, codependency issues
CV 5	*Sea of Intimacy*				
CV 6	*Sea of Energy*				
CV 12	*Center of Power*	On the front midline of the upper abdomen, between the navel and the breastbone	Promotes good digestion; balances appetite; holds overall body tension and stress	Relieves abdominal distension and pain, gastritis, indigestion, ulcers, stomachache, diarrhea, hiccups	Releases stored emotional pain related to abandonment, self-esteem, and boundary issues, anger, shame, guilt, codependency
CV 13	*Upper Channel*				

FEET POINTS

Point #	Point Name	Point Location	Point Function	Physical Imbalances	Emotional & Spiritual Aspects
Sp 1	*Hidden Clarity*	At the medial angle of the base of the big toenail	Regulates the spleen and facilitates blood flow; balances excessive thinking and clears the brain	Relieves dream-disturbed sleep, appetite imbalances, abdominal distension, prolonged menstruation, nausea	Relieves depression, melancholia, worry, mood swings, shock, self-abuse, codependency, abandonment
Sp 3 Sp 4	*Spleen Source* *Grandparent Grandchild*	In the upper arch of the foot, next to ball of the foot (Sp 3); One thumb-width from ball of foot (Sp 4)	Regulates the stomach and spleen; transforms dampness; invigorates digestion	Relieves foot cramp, cold feet, PMS, endometriosis, lower abdominal pain, bloating, indigestion, nausea	Calms restlessness and restores the spirit; relieves abandonment and self-abuse disorders; supports emotional stability
K 3 K 6	*Bigger Stream* *Great Ravine*	In back of the ankle between the inside anklebone and Achilles tendon; Below the inner ankle bone	Balances the kidneys; strengthens the brain; Regulates the andle and energy flow	Relieves swollen feet, backaches, sexual problems, ankle pain, chronic fatigue, labor pain, impotence	Balances fear issues; stabilizes intimate relationships; relieves abandonment feelings, guilt, and incest

KNEE POINTS

Point #	Point Name	Point Location	Point Function	Physical Imbalances	Emotional & Spiritual Aspects
Sp 9 K 10 Sp 10	*Emotional Side of the Mountain* *Yin Valley* *Sea of Blood*	On the inside of the leg below the head of the tibia; At the medial end of the knee crease; Three finger-widths above the kneecap	Regulates the spleen and stomach, resolves dampness; promotes urination and regulates the body's water pathways; governs the production of blood cells	Relieves knee problems, swelling, varicose veins, edema, water retention, atrophy, abdominal distension, genital pain, vaginal discharge, menstrual problems	Nourishes the spirit; emotional shock absorber; relieves worry, mood swings, codependency and boundary issues, fear and phobia; provides emotional support

BACK RELEASE POINTS

Point #	Point Name	Point Location	Point Function	Physical Imbalances	Emotional & Spiritual Aspects
B 42	*Soul Door*	Two finger-widths below the shoulder blade, on the ropy muscles	Governs the strength of the spine; anal and genital functions	Hemorrhoid, anal and genital pain, spinal pain, urinary problems	Chronic insecurity, paranoia, phobia, fear, survival issues, unable to be alone
GV 4	*Gate of Life*	On the lower back between two vertebrae level with the navel	Stabilizes the kidneys; clears the brain; benefits the lower back	Relieves lower back pain; migraine headache, dizziness, painful joints, urinary incontinence	Source of essence; calms the spirit; relieves disorientation, forgetfulness, fear, terror, nightmares
B 23 B 47	*Sea of Vitality Points*	In the lower back, two and four fingers out from the spine, level with the navel	Benefits the kidneys and bladder; supports healing within the body; restores sexual vitality	Relieves exhaustion, fatigue, infertility, lower backache, impotence, lumbago, abdominal disorders	Governs emotional stamina and spiritual renewal; releases fear, phobia, trauma, emotional numbness, anger, depression, withdrawal
B 48	*Womb & Vitals*	Two finger-widths outside the sacrum (at the base of the spine)	Governs the pelvic area; regulates menstruation	Relieves hip pain, PMS, pelvic tension, lower backache, menstrual cramp, sciatica	Frustration, emotional uptightness, rage, resentment, insecurity
B 27– B 34	*Sacral Points*	Base of spine, in the hollows of the bone	Strengthens the lower back; benefits kidney and bladder	Relieves hip pain, sacral pain, lower back pain, and sciatica	Sacred spiritual base; relieves fear
B 54	*Commanding Middle*	In the center of the knee crease in back of the knee	Equalizes energy flow through the back and the back of the legs; stabilizes the knee	Relieves back pain, sciatica, knee pain, arthritis in the knee, back stiffness	Fear, phobia, emotional support, insecurity, self-doubt
GV 1	*Backbone Strength*	At the bottom tip of the tailbone	Governs the mid back, liver, and diaphragm muscles	Relieves digestive disorder, stomach-aches, rib and mid back pain	Anger, resentment, rage, uptightness, numbness, trauma

— POINTS ON THE SIDE OF THE BODY —

Point #	Point Name	Point Location	Point Function	Physical Imbalances	Emotional & Spiritual Aspects
GV 19 GV 20 GV 21	*One Hundred Meeting*	On the top of the back of the head, in hollow on the midline	Clears the brain; good for memory and concentration	Relieves hot flashes, heatstroke, headache, hay fever, epilepsy	Calms the spirit; relieves depression, anxiety, emotional shock and trauma
LI 14	*Upper Arm Bone*	On the outer upper arm, one-third down from top of shoulder to elbow	Governs the upper arm; releases shoulder pain	Relieves aching in the arms, chronic fatigue, fibromyalgia, shoulder tension, stiff neck, toothaches	Guardian of the spirit; relieves melancholy, mood swings, apathy, depression, uptightness
LI 11	*Crooked Pond*	On the outer end of the elbow crease	Strengthens the upper portion of the body; clears the colon; antidepressant	Chronic fatigue, fibromyalgia, weakness, carpal tunnel syndrome	Sadness, depression, overwhelm, mood swings, apathy, melancholy
TW 5	*Outer Gate*	Two finger-widths above the center of the outer wrist crease, between the two bones	Regulates and strengthens the entire body; benefits the immune system	Relieves rheumatism, tendinitis, wrist pain, resistance to cold, flu, fever, chill, nausea, hypertension, shoulder pain, neck stiffness	For emotional projection, reduces vulnerability; relieves depression, sadness, withdrawal, grief
LI 4	*Joining the Valley ("Hoku")*	In the webbing between the thumb and index finger	Balances the gastrointestinal system; alleviates pain in general; anti-inflammatory point	Relieves frontal headache, allergic reaction, constipation, neck and shoulder pain, arthritis, labor pain, hay fever, sinus pain	Valley of hope and spirit; relieves anger, depression, numbness, emotional holding

Appendix B:
Point Location Charts

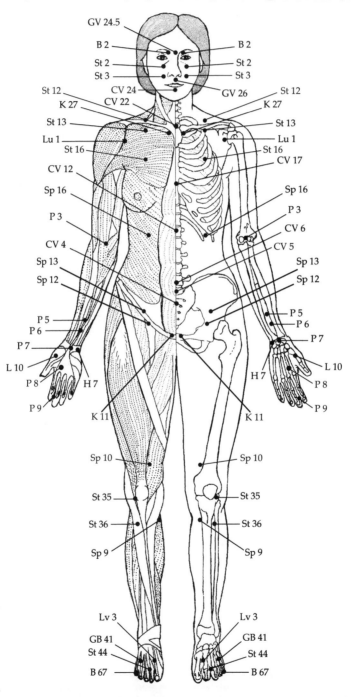

GV 24.5

B 2   B 2
St 2   St 2
St 3   St 3

St 12   CV 24   GV 26   St 12
K 27   CV 22
St 13   K 27
Lu 1   St 13
St 16   Lu 1
                           St 16
CV 12   CV 17

Sp 16   Sp 16

P 3   P 3
                           CV 6
CV 4   CV 5
Sp 13   Sp 13
Sp 12   Sp 12

P 5   P 5
P 6   P 6
P 7   P 7
L 10   L 10
P 8   H 7   H 7 P 8
P 9   P 9

K 11   K 11

Sp 10   Sp 10

St 35   St 35
St 36   St 36
Sp 9   Sp 9

Lv 3   Lv 3
GB 41   GB 41
St 44   St 44
B 67   B 67

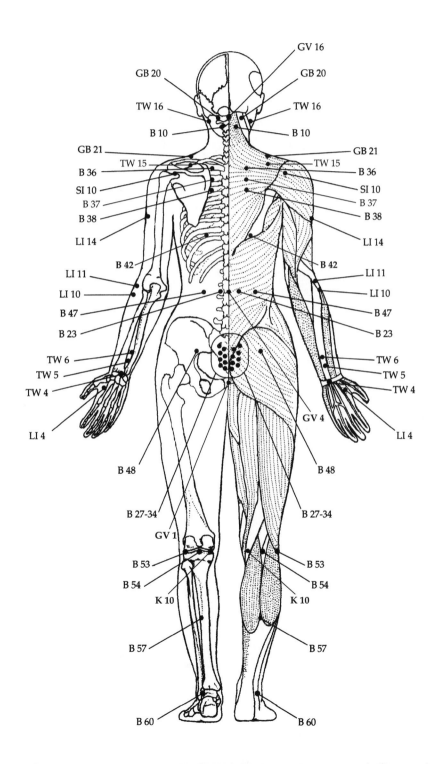

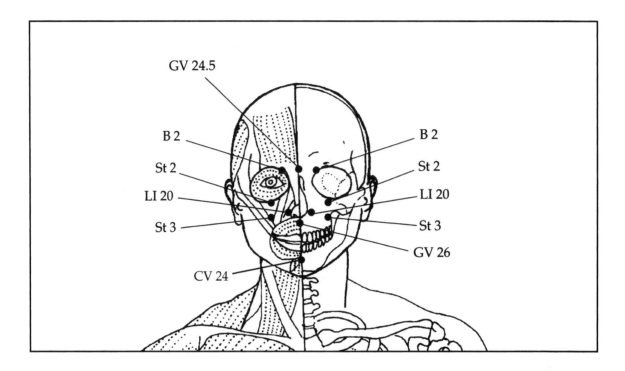

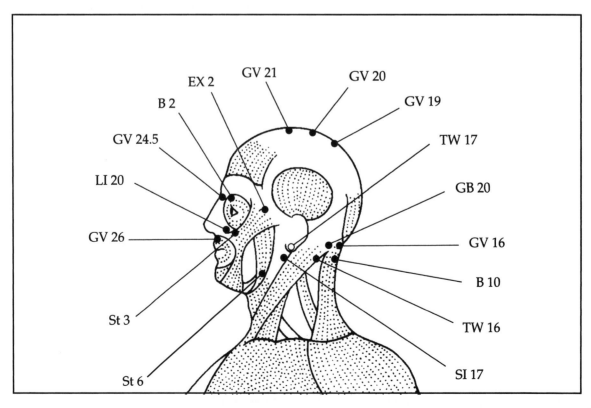

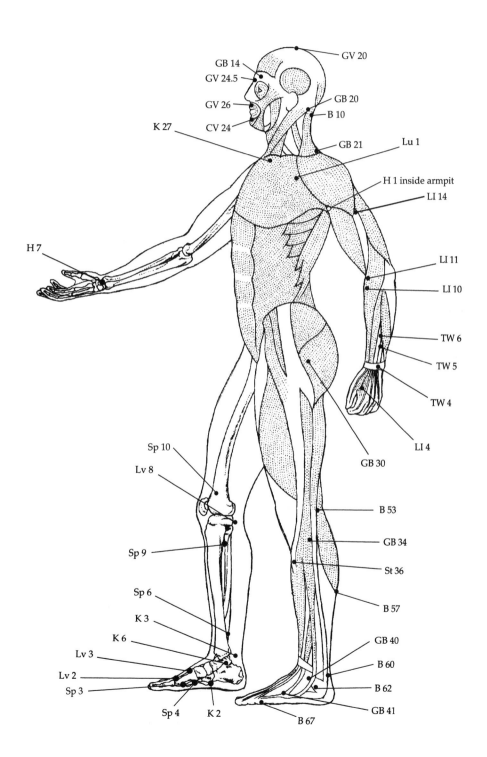

APPENDIX C:
CHAPTER LOG OF POINTS

Abandonment: CV 6, K 27, Lu 1, Sp 16, St 16, St 36

Addiction: CV 12–CV 17, GB 14, GB 20, GB 21, GV 1, GV 16, GV 24.5, K 6, Lv 3, Sp 3, Sp 12, Sp 13, Sp 16, St 16, TW 15

Anger: B 10, B 23, B 47, CV 12, CV 17, GB 20, GB 21, GV 20, P 6, P 9, Sp 12, Sp 13

Anxiety & Panic Attacks: B 23, B 38, B 47, CV 4, CV 5, CV 6, CV 17, GV 24.5, H 7, Lu 1, P 6, P 7

Chronic Fatigue & Fibromyalgia: B 23, B 47, CV 6, CV 17, GV 24.5, LI 4, LI 11, P 6, St 36, TW 5

Codependency: CV 6, CV 12, CV 17, GV 4, GV 20, GV 24.5, P 6

Diet for Emotional Healing: B 23, B 47, CV 6, CV 12, CV 17, GV 20, GV 24.5, GV 26, LI 4, LI 11, Sp 10, Sp 16, St 3, St 16, St 36

Depression: B 10, B 36–B 38, B 47, B 48–B 54, CV 17, GB 14, GB 21, GV 24.5, LI 14, Lu 1, St 36

Emotional Numbness: B 36–B 40, CV 4–CV 14, GB 21

Emotional Support: CV 17, GV 26, Lu 1, St 36

Fear & Phobias: B 23, B 42, B 47, B 62, CV 6, CV 17, GB 14, GV 24.5, K 6, K 27, Lu 1, St 16, St 36

Grief: B 15, B 38, CV 6, CV 12, CV 17, GB 20, GB 21, GB 34, GV 4, LI 11, Lu 1, P 2, P 6, P 8, SI 11, Sp 10, St 36, TW 5, TW 15

Guilt & Shame: B 10, B 23, B 47, CV 6, CV 12, CV 17, CV 24, GB 20, GB 41, GV 16, GV 24.5, K 27, Lu 1, Lv 1, Lv 3, Sp 1, Sp 12, Sp 13, Sp 16, St 35, St 36, St 43, St 45

Incest: B 48, CV 1, CV 6, CV 17, GB 20, H 1, K 27, Lu 1, P 6, Sp 9, Sp 12, Sp 13,

Insomnia: B 10, B 38, B 62, CV 6, CV 12, CV 17, GB 20, GV 16, GV 24.5, H 1, H 7, K 6, K 27, P 6, TW 5

Jealousy & Resentment: CV 6, CV 12, K 27, Lu 1, St 3, St 6

Menstruation & Menopause: B 10, B 27–B 34, B 47, B 48, B 60, CV 6, CV 17, GB 20, GB 21, GB 34, GB 41, GV 4, GV 16, GV 20, GV 24.5, GV 26, H 1, K 3, K 27, LI 4, Lu 1, P 6, SI 10, Sp 4, Sp 6, Sp 9, Sp 10, Sp 12, Sp 13, Sp 16, St 36, TW 15

Mood Swings: CV 6, CV 17, CV 24, GV 24.5, GV 26, K 27, Lv 1, Lv 3, P 6, Sp 1, Sp 3, Sp 4, Sp 12, Sp 13, Sp 16, St 36, TW 5

Nightmares: B 47, CV 6, CV 17, GB 14, GB 20, GV 20, GV 24.5, LI 4, Lu 9, P 6, P 7, St 36, TW 15

Stress & the Emotions: CV 17, GB 20, GB 21, GV 24.5, St 6

Sexual Abuse: CV 4, CV 6, CV 17, GB 20, GV 24.5, H 1, K 11, Sp 12, Sp 13, Sp 16, St 16, St 30

Spirit of the Emotions: B 10, B 23, B 47, CV 6, CV 17, GB 20, GB 21, GV 20, GV 24.5, K 24–K 27, Lu 1, Sp 1, Sp 4, Sp 16, St 13, St 36

Trauma & Post-Traumatic Stress Disorder: B 10, B 27–B 34, CV 6, CV 17, GB 14, GB 20, GB 21, GV 16, GV 24.5, GV 26, K 26, K 27, Lu 1, P 6, P 8, P 9, SI 10, St 12, St 13, St 36, TW 5

Worry & Self-Doubt: B 10, CV 6, CV 12, CV 17, GB 14, GV 16, GV 20, GV 26, Lu 1, Sp 16, St 3, St 36

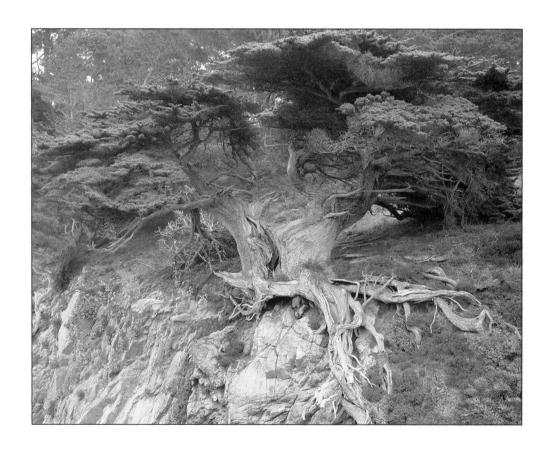

APPENDIX D:

RESOURCES FOR EMOTIONAL HEALING

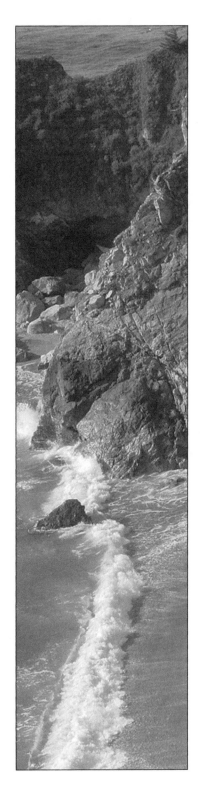

CERTIFIED TRAININGS

Acupressure Institute

The Acupressure Institute in Berkeley, California, established in 1976 by Michael Reed Gach, PhD, offers year-round training programs in traditional Asian bodywork, acupressure, shiatsu, Acu-Yoga teacher training, and therapeutic massage. Students begin with the 150-hour Basic Program and can continue with the 200-hour Emotional Balancing Specialization Program or the 850-hour Acupressure Therapy Program. This unique training teaches the most appropriate points and meridians for healing various emotional problems and imbalances. Learn to incorporate effective counseling skills with acupressure point formulas for relieving trauma, panic attacks, anxiety, post-traumatic stress, depression, phobia, sexual abuse, grief, excessive worry, overwhelming emotions, and more. The Acupressure Institute also has trainings in women's health issues, sports acupressure, pain relief, elder care, and Asian traditional therapies in preparation for the national test in Asian Bodywork Therapy.

Acupressure Institute
1533 Shattuck Avenue
Berkeley, CA 94709
(800) 442-2232
www.acupressure.com

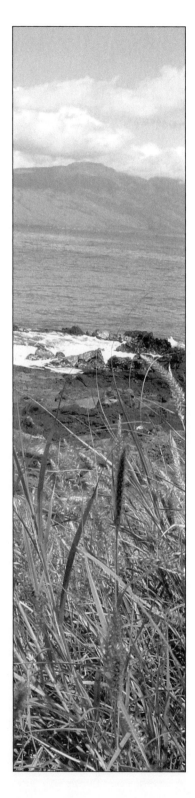

Tao Institute

The Tao Institute, in St. Cloud, Minnesota, offers year-round programming in acupressure and integrated massage styles, Reiki, Shazen somatic therapies, and yoga teacher training, emotional and spiritual balancing, and equine and animal acupressure massage. Classes are limited to offer apprenticeship-style trainings, which are completed within four months to three years. In the 150-hour basic training students learn their foundation in traditional Chinese health care theory and application, hand techniques, and massage rhythms. The 250- and 750-hour advanced programs focus on emotional and spiritual balancing, self-cultivation practices, counseling skills, and advanced esoteric theory and practice. Shazen yogic and somatic practices are designed to increase wellness and support the spiritual balancing process. The 300-hour Animal Acupressure Massage Program offers the opportunity to study traditional Chinese theory, anatomy, acupressure points, meridians, massage styles, and dietary practices.

Tao Institute
223 Seventh Avenue South
St. Cloud, MN 56301
(320) 253-8028
www.taoinstituteinc.com

Asian Bodywork Practitioner Directory

The American Organization for Bodywork Therapies of Asia (AOBTA) publishes the National Asian Bodywork Practitioner Directory, an annual directory of teachers and practitioners of Asian bodywork, including acupressure and shiatsu practitioners. For a quarterly newsletter, information on annual conferences, or a practitioner directory, contact:

AOBTA Headquarters
1010 Haddonfield-Berlin Road, Suite 408
Voorhees, NJ 08043
(856) 782-1616
www.aobta.org

EMOTIONAL HEALING
WORKSHOPS & TRAININGS

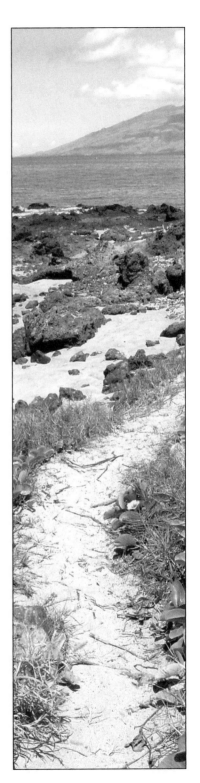

Authors Michael Gach and Beth Henning are excellent, inspiring teachers who combine a friendly, warm, accessible teaching style with precise technical skill. Through their combined forty years of experience, they have discovered groundbreaking healing techniques that have brought pain relief and healing to thousands of people. Beth and Michael are available to teach together or independently. To sponsor a workshop or training in your area contact:

Michael Reed Gach
Acupressure Institute
1533 Shattuck Avenue
Berkeley, CA 94709
(800) 442-2232
gach@acupressure.com

Beth Henning
Tao Institute
223 Seventh Avenue South
St. Cloud, MN 56301
(320) 253-8028
beth@taoinstituteinc.com

Re-Evaluation Co-Counseling

Joining a co-counseling group is a safe, inexpensive way to process emotional distress, resentment, and other unfinished feelings. These groups teach supportive active listening and can be an effective way to release your emotions. For more information and to find a co-counseling group in your area, contact:

Re-Evaluation Counseling Communities
719 Second Avenue North
Seattle, WA 98109
(206) 284-0311
www.rc.org

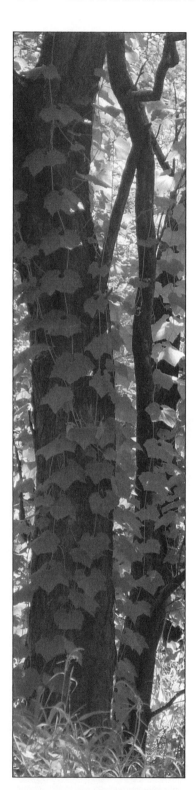

HANDS-ON HEALTH CARE
MAIL-ORDER CATALOG

The Acupressure Institute publishes a mail-order catalog containing a wide variety of materials that can support your personal healing, and show you how to use acupressure to relieve common ailments and enhance your life. The catalog contains:

- Self-Acupressure Books
- Guided Self-Healing CDs
- Magnets & Body Tools
- Lovers Sacred Touch Videos
- Charts, Tapes & Booklets
- Healing Music

Online Store:
www.StressReliefProducts.com

All of the books, charts, CDs, and videos in the catalog are available to order online. You will find self-healing and instructional videos on acupressure, Thai massage, Acu-Yoga, and shiatsu.

Home Study Starter Package:

Michael Reed Gach, PhD, internationally renowned writer, makes learning acupressure easy; there is no testing and the Starter Package is not considered a course. The following products present the basics of acupressure:

- *Acupressure's Potent Points* Book
- *Fundamentals of Acupressure* Video
- *Basic Acupressure Workbook* with point formulas
- *Stress Relief* CD & Acupressure Point Flash Cards
- Acupressure Point Reference Chart:
  A color-coded illustration of the meridians and special points shown from front, back, and side views of the body. Laminated for durability. Size: 24" x 36". Included with the chart is a 16-page Acupressure Point Recipes booklet for common ailments.

All of these products can be ordered separately.

(510) 845-1059
www.StressReliefProducts.com

GLOSSARY

Acupressure: An ancient healing art that uses finger pressure on the acupuncture points and meridians to release muscular pain and tensions and to increase circulation in the body.

Acupuncture: An ancient healing art that inserts fine needles into the body at points to relieve pain and treat various ailments.

Acu-Yoga: A healing art that uses full-body postures along with deep breathing to stretch muscles, open the meridians, and stimulate the acupressure points for self-healing. *See* Yoga.

Affirmation: A positive statement that acknowledges life, that is repeated silently or said aloud. Affirmations reinforce the power of positive thinking.

Blockage: Body congestion causing an ache, tension, pain, and numbness.

Breathing Visualization: A visualization that uses the power of concentration to direct long, deep breaths into specific areas of the body for healing purposes. *See* Visualization.

Centering: The practice of focusing your attention on your body or breathing to become more aware of the present moment.

Chakra: A vital center of life energy based on a major nerve plexus. Each chakra governs specific physical body functions as well as emotional and psychological aspects of a person.

Chi: In traditional Chinese medicine, energy that circulates through meridians. *See* Energy.

Chronic Tension: A long-term contracted muscular condition.

Dissociation: A split in consciousness in which a person feels separate or removed from reality, body awareness, or emotions.

Distal Point: An acupressure point located a distance away from the area it benefits. *See also* Local Point.

Energy: The basis of all life-forms and matter in the universe; a dynamic force that circulates through the body in the meridians.

Five Elements: In traditional Chinese medicine, a major theory that links the properties of wood, fire, earth, water, and metal to the body's senses, tastes, emotions, and fluids, and the functions of the internal organs.

Focusing: The process of guiding awareness within the body by placing your attention on an emotion or body sensation, then exploring what your body is expressing and the inner world of your body's wisdom.

Hara: In Japanese, the vital energy center in the lower abdominal region (*dantien*). The center of the *hara* is CV 6, three finger-widths below the navel, called the Sea of Energy.

Homeostasis: The state of equilibrium or balance within the body.

Intuition: Inner guidance from thoughts and images that create an imminent knowingness.

Lateral: Toward the outside of the body.

Life Force: The vital energy or *chi* contained in all things that circulates through the meridians. *See Chi;* Energy.

Local Point: An acupressure point located in the area it benefits. *See also* Distal Point.

Lumbar Vertebrae: The five large bones of the spine in the lower back above the sacrum.

Medial: Toward the center of the body.

Meditation: Specific mental focusing techniques used to clear and develop the mind.

Meridian: An energy pathway in the body that connects the acupressure points with the internal organs, endocrine glands, lymph, blood, muscles, and nerves.

Meridian Abbreviations:

Listed in the sequence in which the meridians flow.

Lu	Lung	P	Pericardium
LI	Large Intestine	TW	Triple Warmer
St	Stomach	GB	Gall Bladder
Sp	Spleen	Lv	Liver
H	Heart	CV	Conception Vessel
SI	Small Intestine	GV	Governing Vessel
B	Bladder	EX	Extra Point
K	Kidney		

Mudra: In Sanskrit, a hand or finger position used during meditation and yoga that transmits healing energy through the meridians.

Post–Traumatic Stress Disorder: The residual effects of a severe trauma that cause stress and other complaints.

Pressure Point: A gateway for healing energy having a high level of electrical conductivity at the surface of the skin or *chi* along a meridian.

Psychotherapy: The practice of treating an individual's problems, conflicts, emotional imbalances, and personal issues through a range of communication skills, counseling skills, psychoanalysis, suggestion, cathartic exercises, and other processes by a professional therapist.

Referred Pain: Pain that originates in one area of the body but is felt in another.

Sabotage: Unconscious behaviors that prevent positive change and growth.

Sacrum: The flat triangular bone in the lower back at the base of the spine.

Sacroiliac: The joint between the top of the hipbone (ilium) and the fused bottom vertebrae (sacrum).

Shiatsu: In Japanese, finger pressure; a bodywork style that stimulates acupressure points using firm, therapeutic pressure.

Somatic: Pertaining to the body.

Thoracic Vertebrae: Consist of the twelve spinal vertebrae below the neck in the upper and middle back.

Traditional Chinese Medicine: A methodology of medicine developed in ancient China that uses a holistic system of diagnosis involving body and face reading, listening, smelling, in-depth questioning, feeling pulses, and palpating points and meridians.

Trigger Point: A specific location on the surface of the skin that, when pressed, relieves tension, pain, or pressure; most trigger points are also acupressure points.

Visualization: Forming images and thoughts to positively direct one's life.

Yoga: An ancient healing practice from India that uses body postures, stretches, breathing techniques, hand positions (*mudras*), and meditation to attain "union" among the body, mind, and spirit.

Selected Bibliograpy

Acupressure & Chinese Medicine

1. Beinfield, Harriet, and Efrem Korngold. *Between Heaven and Earth: A Guide to Chinese Medicine.* New York: Ballantine Wellspring,1991.

2. Eisenberg, David. *Encounters With Qi.* New York: Norton, 1985.

3. Gach, Michael Reed. *Acupressure's Potent Points.* New York: Bantam Books, 1990.

4. Gach, Michael Reed. *Acupressure for Lovers.* New York: Bantam Books, 1996.

5. Hammer, Leon, MD. *Dragon Rises, Red Bird Flies.* New York: Station Hill Press, 1990.

6. Kaptchuk, Ted J. *The Web That Has No Weaver.* New York: Congdon & Weed, 1983.

7. Pitchford, Paul. *Healing with Whole Foods.* Berkeley, CA: North Atlantic Books, 1993.

8. Teeguarden, Iona Marsaa. *Acupressure Way of Health.* New York: Japan Publications, 1978.

Emotional Healing

1. Adams, Kathleen. *Journal to the Self: 22 Paths to Personal Growth.* New York: Warner Books, 1990.

2. Bass, Ellen and Laura Davis. *The Courage to Heal: A Guide for Women Survivors of Child Sexual Abuse.* New York: HarperCollins, 1992.

3. Branden, Nathaniel. *If You Could Hear What I Cannot Say.* New York: Bantam Doubleday Dell, 1983.

4. Davis, Laura. *The Courage to Heal Workbook.* New York: HarperCollins, 1990.

5. Gendlin, Eugene T. *Focusing.* New York: Bantam New Age Books, 1981.

6. Hendricks, Gay, and Kathlyn Hendricks. *At The Speed of Life: A New Approach to Personal Change Through Body-Centered Therapy.* New York: Bantam Books, 1994.

7. Ruskan, John. *Emotional Clearing.* New York: R. Wyler, 1993.

8. Padus, Emrika. *The Complete Guide to Your Emotions and Your Health.* Emmaus, PA: Rodale Press, 1992.

Spirituality

1. Dalai Lama. *The Art of Happiness.* New York: Riverhead Books, 1998.

2. Hanh, Thich Nhat. *Transformation and Healing.* Berkeley, CA: Parallax Press, 1990.

3. Hanh, Thich Nhat. *Teachings on Love.* Berkeley, CA: Parallax Press, 1998.

4. Hanh, Thich Nhat. *Anger: Wisdom for Cooking the Flames.* New York: Riverhead Books, 2001.

5. Ruiz, Don Miguel. *The Mastery of Love.* San Rafael, CA: Amber-Allen, 1999.

6. Zukav, Gary. *The Seat of the Soul.* New York: Simon & Schuster, 1989.

Acknowledgments

We are grateful for the ancient teachings and to all our teachers who have contributed to our growth and knowledge. Tremendous appreciation goes out to our loving parents, who through example gave us emotional depth.

Many people gave us personal support and guidance while we were writing this book. We especially want to thank the staff and students at our schools—the Acupressure Institute in Berkeley, California, and the Tao Institute in St. Cloud, Minnesota—for supporting us to teach this wonderful hands-on healing information.

Barbara Terrill Gach's significant contribution to this book—her understanding of alternative and complementary health practices, her editing and writing skills, her insights, and her spiritual depth—deserves special acknowledgment. Much of the clarity and accessibility of this book is due to her suggestions and feedback.

We would like to express our appreciation to Zachary and Ayriel Steffes, Beth's children, for their mindfulness, patience, love, and understanding of time constraints, throughout the six years of this book project.

Judi Newville at Inner Peace Books deserves special acknowledgment for her understanding of emotional and spiritual balancing, her patience in rearranging clientele, her editing input, and her friendship.

Kathleen Farrell, James Henning, Patricia Kleindl, Dale Zimmerman, Peggy LaDou, Dr. Jeffrey Varner, James Steffes, Dr. George Schoephoester, Kaya, Kathryn Edwards, and Brad and Mary Dean Johnson deserve special recognition for their editing feedback, professional expertise, or personal friendship and guidance.

Great appreciation goes to our editor, Philip Rappaport, who gave us a comprehensive critique of the manuscript along with numerous outstanding suggestions for improving it. His insightful, articulate input inspired our creativity and expanded the scope of this book. We would also like to thank Toni Burbank for her support, insight, and wise consultation.

We are grateful for the following psychotherapists and colleagues who offered their professional advice, editorial feedback, and guidance: Bridget Simmerman, LCSW; Jean Hayek, MA, MFT; Karen O'Conner, MA; Meg Flynn, MA, MFT; James Bryer, MA, MFT; Michael Mayer, PhD; Anthony Luzi; Paul Abell, PhD; and Michael Blondeau Gelbart, MSW, ACSW, LCS. We appreciate Joseph Carter, LAc, for reviewing the point location accuracy on the anatomical drawings.

Karin Kinsey from Dolphin Press did an outstanding job producing the graphics and book design. David Lehrer shot all of the fine photographs in the book. We would also like to acknowledge the models in the book: Janiece Piper, Edward Spencer, Asha Romero, Barbara Marienthal, Olivia Ford, Thin Thin Yu, and Carlos Castillo. Special thanks to Lela Davia, who helped direct the models during the photo shoot.

CLOSING
AFFIRMATIONS

I can change my world
By letting go of my expectations
Returning to the present moment.

I can change my world
By breathing deeply,
Appreciating who I am,
Accepting instead of judging
All that I have in my life,
And what is right here before me.

I can change my world,
By holding points to heal myself;
Listening to my body's perceptions—
Making sense of its thoughts and feelings,
Trusting the depths of my emotions
In guiding me to nurture my spirit.

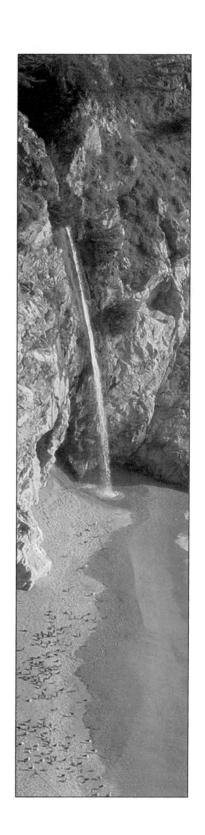

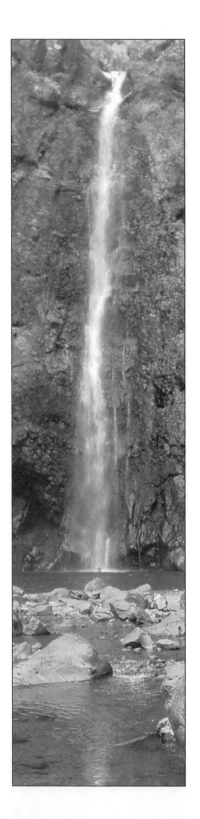

Concluding
Supportive Notes

Keep your healing intentions and faith alive.
Be patient with your emotional healing process,
Don't let obstacles or your pain discourage you.

Embrace what is difficult; learn from these tests,
Letting the challenges empower you instead.
Perseverance furthers emotional healing.

Listen to your body's wisdom
And continue to breathe deeply.
Each deep breath you take
Nourishes your body and spirit,
Cultivating an inner awareness—
Your intuition to know what is right

Emotions are the jewels of being human.
Tears not only express emotional pain;
They also awaken the depths of your heart.
Each emotional healing experience
Brings you closer to setting you
Free from the past, forever…

INDEX

Y